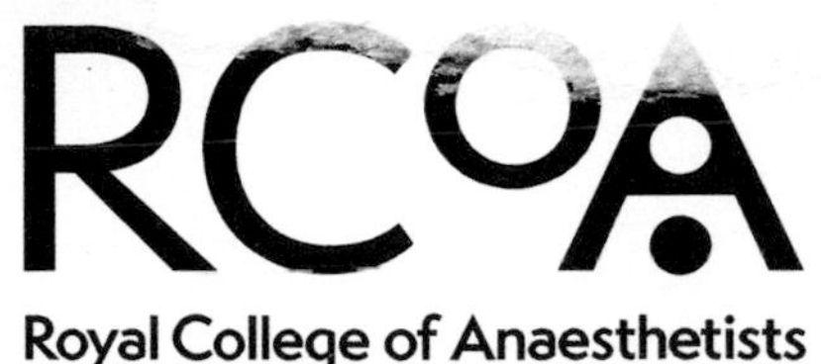

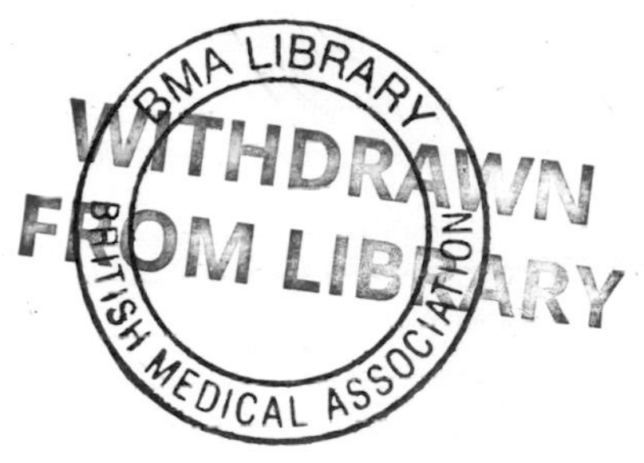

Guide to the FRCA examination
The Primary

Fourth Edition
December 2013

Editor
Dr Mike Wilkinson

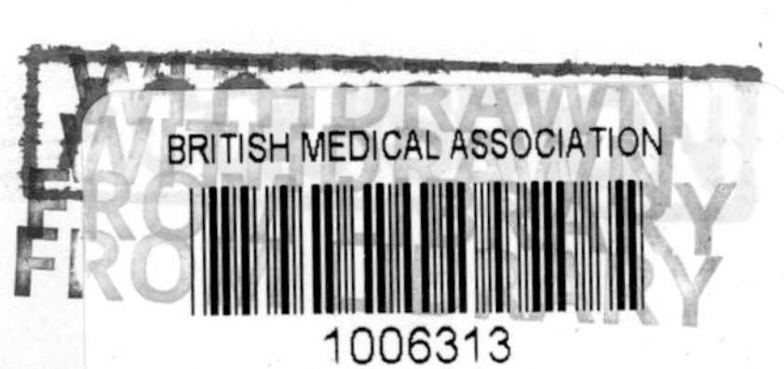

ISBN 978-1-900936-22-4

Disclaimer

This Guide and any content, information, texts, images and graphics provided thereon ('Content') are provided to you by the Royal College of Anaesthetists, and the Content authors on the following basis:

The Guide and Content are provided on an 'as is' basis. To the fullest extent permitted by law, we give no guarantees, warranties, representations, endorsements, express, implied or statutory, with regard to the Guide or the Content, including without limitation the information presented in this Guide concerning medical procedures, drug doses and their application. The Content does not constitute any form of advice or recommendation by us and is not intended to be relied upon in making (or refraining from making) any specific medical or other decisions. All users should consult other medical literature to determine the correct procedures, the correct drug doses and their correct application for each individual patient.

To the fullest extent permitted by law, we shall not be liable to you (whether in contract, tort, negligence or otherwise) for any loss or damage of any nature whether direct, indirect or consequential and arising out of or in connection with this Guide whether due to omission, error or inaccuracy or any other cause and whether on our part or that of our servants, agents or any other person.

You shall fully indemnify us for and against all and any losses, costs (including without limitation any legal costs on a full indemnity basis), damages, claims and liabilities suffered or incurred by us as a result of any third party claim against us arising from your use of the Guide.

English law shall govern the access to and use of this Guide and its Content.

Design and layout by the Royal College of Anaesthetists

Contents

Section 3: Answers and guidance

Introduction

The Council of the Royal College of Anaesthetists agreed in 2001 that some of the material used in the examinations for the Diploma of Fellow of the Royal College of Anaesthetists should be made available in order to help candidates in their exam preparation. As a result of this, the first Guide to the Primary examination was published, with two revised editions published in 2007 and 2010 taking into account the changes in the delivery and conduct of the examination determined by the Postgraduate Medical Education and Training Board (PMETB) in 2005 and 2009. Further changes to the exam in line with the requirements of the GMC have now been instituted requiring a fourth revision of the guide.

This publication was never intended to be a textbook, but rather a guide to the examination process and to aid candidates in their studies. All information regarding the format and conduct of the examination is correct at the date of publication. Exam changes, once approved by Council are published in the College *Bulletin* and the *Candidate* Newsletter, information updates and candidate resources for examinations which include video and question examples are available on the examinations pages on the College website (www.rcoa.ac.uk). This book, which covers the Primary FRCA examination, is divided along the same lines as the examination itself. There are examples of multiple-choice questions (MCQs) – taken from the College MCQ bank – with answers and brief explanations. The section on the structured oral examination (SOE) is illustrated with examples from the current examination material and includes the guidance given to examiners regarding the subject areas to be covered. The objective structured clinical examination (OSCE) question examples are also included, again with some material currently in use.

All the questions have been checked by examiners against a variety of sources and mapped to the Basic Level Training curriculum of the CCT in Anaesthesia. Every effort has been made to ensure that the answers given are correct but there may be differences of opinion at times and no responsibility can be accepted by the College for any errors. Developing new questions takes a considerable amount of time and effort by many examiners and I thank not only those responsible for the material in this book but also all examiners for their unstinting support and contribution to the development of the exam. It is the hope of the Council of the College, and of the examiners, that candidates and their trainers, will find this fourth edition of the guide helpful and useful.

Dr Mike Wilkinson
Chairman – Primary FRCA Examination

ABOUT THE EXAMINATION

1

Scoring and assessment

The Primary FRCA examination is divided into three sections, a multiple choice question (MCQ) written exam, an objective structured clinical exam (OSCE) and a structured oral exam (SOE). Each section independently has a pass or fail outcome based upon an aggregate score. To achieve an overall pass in the Primary, a candidate must pass **all three** sections.

The MCQ paper is a stand-alone written examination, applied for independently of the OSCE/SOE, and must be passed before a candidate can apply to sit the OSCE/SOE components. A pass in the MCQ section may be retained for a maximum of three years. This section has recently changed to include single best answer (SBA) questions, a full explanation of this and the MCQ as a whole is given in the MCQ section.

Following success in the MCQ a candidate is eligible to enter the OSCE/SOE sections of the exam. A candidate may choose which sitting of the exam they wish to enter. However, at the first attempt both the OSCE and SOE must be taken together. If a candidate passes one section but fails the other then they may re-enter for the failed section only. If both sections are failed then the next attempt must include both the OSCE and SOE sections. A pass in either section remains valid for two years. A reduced fee is payable by a candidate sitting only one section.

During the OSCE and SOE sections no examiner has knowledge of a candidate's performance in any previous attempts. Neither do they have knowledge of their performance on any particular day, so candidates should not be concerned that any performance issues in one area would affect their chances elsewhere in the exam.

The standard used to determine a pass is that of a level of knowledge and competence appropriate for a year two trainee (CT2). There is no 'quota' of passing candidates; all candidates reaching the required standard will pass the exam. A robust quality assurance process exists to ensure that the chance of a candidate passing, on any particular day or sitting, is roughly the same despite the multiple variables that exist.

Candidates should prepare thoroughly for this exam. It is challenging and covers a broad syllabus. Most candidates prepare well for the MCQ and practise many hundreds of questions. This helps considerably to improve their chance of success. The MCQs in this book are drawn from the College question bank and show the range and content of material examined. There are many more questions in the bank and they are revised on a regular basis by the MCQ core group.

It is important that the same meticulous preparation goes in to the oral exams. If you attend for the day poorly prepared and with little knowledge of what is required you will not do yourself justice. The oral exams require certain skills to be practised and the earlier you start to do this the better you will be when you present for the exam. For the OSCE try to practise the key aspects of performance for each station and try to attend at least one full practice round of OSCE. It is hard work and tiring to complete 17 or 18 stations in a row and prior experience of this will help. For the SOE practise answering questions under exam conditions, allowing five minutes for each question. Make sure you explain concepts in depth showing clear thinking and understanding. Try to practise with your tutors and educational supervisors, they will have some knowledge of the exam process and will be able to help guide you.

This Guide should help candidates with their preparation, and tutors and clinical supervisors in their advice. The questions are illustrative, not comprehensive. The structured oral examination questions used in this book reflect recent changes in the structure of the oral examination to ensure that all candidates are given the maximum opportunity to show the depth and breadth of their knowledge. The intention is to help candidates understand and appreciate what they will be faced with in the examination proper. It is for this reason that the SOE answers are succinct. They are guides to the content of the answers and should be used as such. Use each section as a template for further learning in your preparation for the examination and to help conduct your pre-examination practice orals in a fashion similar to the actual event.

Dr Mike Wilkinson

Dr Jane Bembridge – Vice Chairman, Primary FRCA Examination

Multiple choice question examination (MCQ)

Format of the MCQ examination and marking scheme

The multiple choice question component of the Primary FRCA examination is fundamentally a test of knowledge of the basic sciences underpinning the practice of anaesthesia. Since September 2011 the MCQ examination has comprised 60 Multiple True False (MTF) and 30 Single Best Answer (SBA) questions. It is held three times per year in March, September and November.

The MTF paper comprises 60 questions divided into three subsections: Pharmacology, Physiology and Physics (including Clinical Measurement and Statistics), covering the entire Basic Level Training curriculum of the CCT in Anaesthesia. Each subsection contains approximately 20 questions. An MTF question has a common stem with five independent 'leaves', each of which may be either true or false. A correct answer scores one mark and an incorrect answer scores zero. The range of scores for any individual question is therefore zero to five and the maximum score for the entire MTF paper is 300 marks. As there is no penalty for an incorrect answer, all questions should be attempted.

The SBA paper comprises 30 questions. Like the MTF paper it is divided into three subsections; Pharmacology, Physiology and Physics (including Physical Measurement and Statistics). However, SBA questions often have an applied clinical context such that an individual question may test knowledge and its understanding or application in more than one domain. An SBA question has a stem, a lead-in and five options. The stem is a statement relating to a basic science topic or clinical scenario. It is important to realise that all the required information to answer the question is provided in the stem, so any information not provided is unnecessary. The lead-in asks a question based on the information given in the stem, usually in the form: 'Which of the following options is the best/most appropriate/safest etc?' All five options are plausible but only one of them is the 'best' answer.

The classically described SBA comprises five options, which are all true statements. However, it is often difficult to write basic science questions that satisfy this condition and SBA questions in the Primary FRCA examination may comprise options, not all of which are true statements. Options often comprise a list of statements or even a single word (e.g. the names of five drugs), which in and of themselves are neither true nor false. Some SBA questions require a calculation, in which case the five options are plausible answers to the calculation but clearly only one is correct.

Each SBA question scores four marks for a correct answer and zero marks for any of the incorrect answers. Although each SBA question has five options, the SBA paper contains only 30 functional questions, and is therefore marked out of 120. The rationale for this SBA marking scheme is that four incorrect leaves must be eliminated by the candidate in order to answer each question correctly. As there is no penalty for an incorrect answer, all questions should be attempted.

Candidates often ask why the established format of the Primary FRCA MCQ examination comprising 90 Multiple True False (MTF) questions, which had performed well over many years and with which candidates were very familiar, was revised to include Single Best Answer (SBA) questions. The initiative was a response to criticisms made by the Postgraduate Medical Education and Training Board (PMETB) that the focus of MTF questions was too narrow and addressed rote knowledge only, rather than the understanding and application of knowledge. The RCoA was challenged to 'modernise' the examination to accord with models of best examining practice, in line with all of the other major UK postgraduate medical examination boards, which had already adopted alternatives to MTF questions, including SBA questions. In this context the Board of Examiners and Council of the RCoA agreed to work towards the introduction of SBA questions as a component of the MCQ examination and to exploit the opportunities that this would present to improve the examination.

Assessment of 'knows how' and 'knows why' rather than simply 'knows' is better assessed by SBA questions and provides the MCQ examination with a new dimension. SBA questions also have the potential to be more discriminatory as the range of candidate marks is generally 20-100%, whereas that for MTF questions is 50-100%.

Validation and Standard Setting

MTF questions are well established and are relatively easy to write – facts are simply either true or false. As SBA questions are new, a process has been developed which allows us to be confident that question setting is as robust as we can make it. As such, the writing and preparation of SBA questions involves many people devoting a considerable amount of time to the process. Questions are written in draft form by Primary FRCA examiners and forwarded to the ten-member MCQ Core Group for further revision. Each finalised SBA question is mapped to the Basic Level Training Curriculum of the

CCT in anaesthesia and at least one reference sought from source material, which should be familiar to candidates ready to progress to ST3 training, for example; standard textbooks, guidelines and protocols of professional bodies (e.g. Resuscitation Council UK, Difficult Airway Society etc.) and e-Learning Anaesthesia. Questions may be piloted before first use by trainees attending revision courses run by the RCoA and by Primary Examiners from outside the MCQ Core Group. The aim of SBA question writing is to produce questions that address important aspects of basic science, discriminate well between candidates of different ability and are well constructed so that the correct SBA option is answered by the largest group of candidates.

Appropriate standard-setting is key. The pass mark for the Primary FRCA MCQ examination is determined by criterion referencing using a modified Angoff process. In essence, this is based on the collective judgement of Core Group members of how likely the 'borderline' pass/fail candidate is to know the answer to each question on a scale of 0-10. The MTF and SBA papers are assessed separately so that an Angoff pass mark is determined for each component. However, there is no requirement to pass each component separately. Thus, the Angoff pass marks for both the MTF and SBA papers are nominal and the overall MCQ examination Angoff pass mark is a summation of the two. A downward adjustment to the Angoff pass mark is then applied to the MCQ examination, equal to the Standard Error of Measurement (SEM). This has been 8-10 marks (approximately 2% of the total examination mark) since September 2011 and is a statistical tool used to allow for the fact that no examination is 100% reliable. Thus, a candidate who fails the examination by one mark, has actually underperformed with respect to the Angoff standard set by examiners by a more significant margin.

The Core Group convenes immediately after each sitting of the examination to evaluate the performance of both candidates and the examination paper itself. Each of the MTF and SBA questions is examined in turn and the Angoff pass mark for the combined paper reduced accordingly for any question where there is evidence of unreliability, i.e. one mark for a single MTF leaf, five marks for a MTF stem and four marks for an SBA question.

Table 1 on the next page summarises the data on candidate performance in the first three MCQ examinations, which included both MTF and SBA questions. It should be noted that the pass mark and pass rate of each component are nominal and for guidance only. The overall pass mark for the MCQ examination is derived using statistical data relevant to the combined examination. It is therefore possible to perform relatively less well in one component and still pass overall by a relatively better performance in the other component.

Table 1: Candidate performance in MCQ examination

	September 2011	February 2012	June 2012
Number of candidates	304	271	493
Overall MCQ examination pass rate (%)	71.4%	55.4%	61.3%
MTF paper			
Candidate mean mark/300 (%)	233.4 (77.8%)	231.8 (77.3%)	237.3 (79.1%)
Angoff pass mark after SEM correction	240	239	237
Nominal pass rate (%)	42.4%	41.3%	55.0%
Range candidate marks (%)	185-280 (61.7-93.3%)	167-276 (55.7-92.0%)	156-286 (52.0-95.3%)
SBA paper			
Candidate mean mark/120 (%)	82.7 (68.9%)	69.9 (58.3%)	65.3 (54.4%)
Angoff pass mark after SEM correction	65	60	60
Nominal pass rate (%)	86.5%	79.0%	71.6%
Range candidate marks (%)	40-120 (33.3-100%)	28-104 (23.3-86.7%)	32-100 (26.7-83.3%)

It is apparent that on each of these three occasions when a combined MTF and SBA paper ran, mean candidate performance in the SBA component exceeded the nominal pass mark (pass rates of 86.5%, 79.0% and 71.6%) whereas mean candidate performance in the MTF component fell short of the nominal pass mark on two out of the three occasions (pass rates of 42.4%, 41.3% and 55.0%). Therefore the impact of adding SBA questions was to increase the overall pass rate in these three examinations. The mean candidate MTF % mark is higher than the mean SBA % mark because guessing MTF questions gains 50% marks on average compared with only 20% by guessing SBA questions. Thus a candidate who fails the MCQ examination should not make the error of simply attributing his or her failure to an SBA % mark being lower than the overall combined % pass mark – the same will also be true of most candidates who pass the MCQ examination.

The specimen MCQ paper in this book contains actual questions taken from the RCoA Primary FRCA question bank. As such it will give candidates preparing to sit the examination a good idea of the standard required. Brief explanations of the reasoning behind the correct answers are also included. In order to be reasonably sure of success, candidates should aim to achieve 80% in the MTF section and 60% in the SBA section.

Dr Anthony McCluskey – Chairman Primary MCQ Core Group

Objective structured clinical examination (OSCE)

Background

OSCEs have been extensively used in undergraduate medical assessments and their use in postgraduate medicine in the UK was pioneered by the RCoA; this model has now been introduced, in modified forms, in most of the postgraduate medical and surgical examinations. As with all sections of the FRCA examination, the performance of a candidate is unknown to the examiners until the results are given at the end of the day. The RCoA OSCE is an examination that involves a circuit of short test stations, with candidates starting at different places and moving round until everyone has completed all stations. Unlike the oral examinations, if a candidate has prior knowledge of an examiner – such as working in the same department, this will not lead to a change in examiner.

Basic Information

The OSCE tests apply knowledge and skills in a variety of clinical areas, with the style of the station varying according to the topic being examined. All the questions cover subjects from the Basic Level Training curriculum and are mapped to it. The questions are also regularly updated to reflect current practice and any new relevant clinical practice guidelines or hazard reports. The process of an OSCE follows clear guidelines; the questions, instructions to candidates and examiners and the marking schedules are specific and fixed, with examiners being unable to influence the outcome in any way.

In each OSCE 'run' there are 17 stations in total, 16 active stations plus one additional trial station which is included to test the standard and functionality of new questions before they are included in the exam. The trial stations are not identified to candidates or examiners and all 17 stations should therefore be regarded as 'active'. Occasionally an 18th station is included as a rest station to facilitate a larger cohort of candidates going through the OSCE on a given day.

A candidate's result in the OSCE is determined from the total of his/her scores in the 16 active stations. All stations are marked out of 20, so the maximum score that can be obtained is 320. Each individual station has a pass mark determined before the examination, using the modified Angoff technique, and these are aggregated to give the overall pass score. This value will vary slightly according to the combination of questions used in a particular OSCE.

Although stations carry equal weight, the weighting of marks for individual questions within a station may vary according to their clinical importance i.e. they may be worth more than one mark. There are no 'killer' stations, in which poor performance at that station results in an automatic fail of the whole OSCE, and indeed it is still possible to have an overall pass even if zero is scored in one station. If a candidate has a 'bad' station, he/she should try to score every mark possible in it, but be reassured that there are more than enough other stations left to gain an overall pass. Continuing to worry about a previous station may well ensure that poor performance also occurs at the next one, and the next one.

There is no negative marking in any station or question in the OSCE. Candidates should therefore attempt to answer all questions, even if they are not certain their answer is correct, especially in the X-ray stations where a True/False style mark sheet is used.

If a candidate is stuck on a question, the examiner should move on to the next one after an appropriate length of time to ensure the candidate is given the best chance of obtaining the pass mark for the station. The examiners are not, however, permitted to go back to an earlier question if the answer was not known or given incorrectly. This is because earlier answers are often identified in the wording of later questions.

The process

There are normally four OSCE 'runs' during each examination day, two in the morning and another two in the afternoon. Each run has the same basic template of 17 mixed stations with the same questions being asked of the two cohorts in the morning. At lunchtime there is a change to a completely different set of questions for the two afternoon cohorts. The candidates cannot interact during the changeover mid-morning or mid-afternoon.

The OSCE takes place on the 1st floor of Churchill House, and after registering in the reception area on the ground floor candidates will be taken to the waiting area on level one. The supervising examiner will ensure that candidates know their starting station number and run through a brief orientation, including a repeat of the main pieces of advice for the conduct of the exam. As in all sections of the examination, candidates are only identified by their candidate number and this should be visible to the examiner to confirm that they have the correct candidate at their station.

Once all is ready, candidates will be led to the examination room to wait by the instruction point at their starting station. After a minute of familiarising themselves with the station, during which an examiner will check that

candidates are at their correct starting station, a bell will go and they should enter the booth to start the station. After five minutes the bell sounds again to signal the end of the station and candidates then move clockwise in order of increasing station number (5 to 6, 6 to 7, 7 to 8, etc.) There is one minute between stations during which the candidate should read the instructions at the information point carefully in order to know what is expected at the next station.

The timing of the OSCE is very tight, and candidates must ensure that they attend in good time for their allocated session.

Actors

The objective nature of the examination precludes the use of individual patients with clinical signs. Where clinical skills are being examined, for instance in taking a history, the consistency of a professional actor is invaluable. The actors should not be expected to have any abnormal clinical signs and it is the approach and method of the candidate that is being tested.

Causing distress or potential harm to the actor, even in a simulated scenario, is an indication of poor technique.

The stations

The questions in the OSCE are developed by specialist sub-groups of examiners, and reviewed carefully before every exam. New questions go through at least two trial runs and a minimum number of candidates to demonstrate satisfactory performance before being adopted into the question bank.

Although there is considerable variation between types of question, candidates are expected to demonstrate certain core skills within each station. For each exam the question mix within the 17 stations is chosen to cover a diversity of subject areas.

Although five minutes is allowed for each station, several may take far less than this to complete. Some stations, however, will take the full five minutes even for the best candidates. When the examiner is 'leading' the station i.e. is asking all the questions, he/she will tell you when you have reached the end of a station early, and may then chat about other things to help you remain calm. For a station where you are pacing events i.e. doing the asking, such as the history and communication stations, if you decide you have completed the station, simply say so to the examiner, and you can relax for the remaining time, though you will not then be able to return to the question.

For stations involving physical contact with actors or equipment, gloves and alcohol gel are available for candidates to use if they so wish. However, this is not an integral part of any station and candidates will not be penalised if they choose not to do so.

Anatomy

There are two anatomy stations, testing all areas relevant to anaesthesia as detailed in the curriculum. This includes the appropriate surface and deep anatomical relationships of important structures, particularly those relating to the safe practice of regional anaesthesia and invasive monitoring.

Stations may use models, pictures, illustrations or volunteers/actors on whom surface anatomy can be described. Prior practice in explaining the anatomy relevant to local anaesthetic techniques is invaluable.

Communication

Communication is a two-way process involving the passage of information and seeking a response to it. In this interactive station, the candidate will be assessed on his/her ability to communicate effectively about a clinical scenario with a simulated patient, relative or staff member. It is essential that you read the pre-station instructions carefully to ensure you know precisely what you have to communicate at this station.

Performing well requires the candidate to identify i) the level of understanding ii) the level of anxiety and iii) the language skills of the simulated character. These stations all have a specific purpose, which is made clear in the information given prior to the station. If that end-point is not reached, marks will probably be lost.

Some of these stations have 'patients' who are upset, angry, frustrated or worried, and marks are given for a calm, considerate yet informative approach. A cavalier or condescending approach is unlikely to be successful in these cases.

Of all the stations, it is the communication one where the candidate will most likely run out of time. The candidate must practise these skills against the clock before attending the OSCE. They may be highly adept at communication, but this must be matched by effective use of time.

X-ray interpretation

There are two X-ray stations in which an X-ray or other radiological images, such as CT scans, are presented on a computer screen. These stations are currently the only elements of the examination without a direct examiner presence, with the candidate completing the mark sheet alone. An invigilator will ensure that an Optical Mark Reader (OMR) answer sheet, with the correct candidate number pre-printed on it, is already in the station for each candidate. The candidate

needs to check that their candidate number correlates with the one on the answer sheet. Pencils and erasers are provided to mark the sheet, so answers can be changed, but the candidate must make sure their final choice is clear for the OMR machine. The X-ray stations are usually completed well within the allotted time, and provide a slight relaxation from the more busy stations.

Equipment

The equipment station requires the candidate to perform a basic safety check on some of the equipment used in routine anaesthetic practice, and answer some questions relating to its use. It may include an anaesthetic machine or breathing system, or any equipment used for management of the airway, fluid administration or neuraxial blockade.

A clear, safe and logical approach is essential to success. There are no tricks and if you find even the most obvious fault simply indicate that this is the case and that you would not therefore be happy to use it.

Even though a specific anaesthetic machine may be unfamiliar, it is the basic generic skills applicable to all machines that will be expected of you, and if you cannot find a specific control knob, indicate to the examiner what you are looking for. Remember that organisations other than the RCoA publish guidelines, for example The Association of Anaesthetists of Great Britain and Ireland, and these can be and are used to formulate OSCE questions in this and other stations. The worrying observation about this station is that routine checking of anaesthetic equipment seems to be unfamiliar for some candidates. Candidates need to be aware, and are reminded at the pre-OSCE briefing, that for safety reasons it is air that is used in the compressor for the anaesthetic machine and the oxygen monitor will always read 21%, this is not a fault.

Hazards

There are many ways in which harm can potentially be done to patients during anaesthesia and surgery and these are tested in the hazard station, along with ways of preventing them. They may relate to equipment used in theatre, the prescribing of drugs used in anaesthetic practice or the physiological problems that can occur in an unconscious patient.

History

The history stations are where candidates can easily go off in the wrong direction and fail to do themselves justice. You must concentrate on eliciting the relevant information which may be connected to past or present events, may be about pre-existing medical or surgical conditions, or be more specifically related to anaesthesia. Marks will be awarded on the ability to obtain the necessary information from the patient in an efficient, clear and polite manner. There are no marks for describing an anaesthetic technique or potential risk.

There are two history stations, each testing your skills in gaining relevant information from a simulated patient during a pre-operative visit. In both you are simply assessed by an examiner in the station while taking the history. Marks can be gained in some of the history stations by asking about the reasons why the patient is having the procedure so it is always worth considering that aspect.

Both stations require a clear, structured approach to the history taking, and a professional and polite attitude to the whole process. Establishing a good rapport with the actor/actress is also likely to help in gaining maximum information in the limited time available. While individual candidates may differ in their approach to the patient, shaking hands for instance, respect for the 'patient' should be apparent at all times. Starting in the academic year 2013-14 a change to the marking scheme for some of the History and Communication stations will be introduced. This will enable the examiner to allocate an increased number of marks to the style and method used by the candidate to obtain information from the patient. Candidates will be expected to demonstrate a structured and logical approach to obtaining a history and in communicating important information to the 'patient'.

Measurement

This is another station where basic science will be tested, and many of the artefacts are diagrammatic or photographic representations of measurement devices or delivery systems. The candidate will be expected to display an understanding of the basic physical principles used, sources of error, clinical applications and limitations of use.

Monitoring

The subjects asked about in the monitoring station overlap with those covered in SOE 2 but the question content is quite different. As well as understanding the scientific principles of function, the candidate may have to demonstrate practical skills in either setting up or calibrating the equipment and identifying common sources of error. This station does not usually involve actors or volunteers, and may be completed rapidly.

Physical examination

The physical examination station requires the candidate to display to the examiner an appropriate method of examination of a body system, for example the respiratory system or the cranial nerves. The candidate should be polite and considerate to the 'patient', and explain what and why they are doing things. Actions should be absolutely clear to the examiner, even if it appears to make the process somewhat exaggerated.

The level required is at least that of a medical student in their first clinical posting, and some candidates may benefit from a revision course from medical clinical skills trainers prior to presenting to the examination. The range of skills encompasses routine medical examination and the assessment of clinical cases, such as following trauma.

Resuscitation

There are two resuscitation stations. They deal with peri-arrest or arrest scenarios which can be theatre or non-theatre based. One will concentrate on the theoretical aspects of management (including recognition of rhythm abnormality), whilst the other will involve the practical management of a scenario using a simulator (see below). The exact nature of an individual station will vary between practical resuscitation skills, more complex decision-making, or a combination. If a defibrillator is required, there will be an examiner or other qualified resuscitation officer to guide you with the operation of the specific machine used. It is a station where it is essential that you read the instructions at the information point very carefully to know exactly what is required.

Although it might be expected that the limited number of types of cardio-respiratory arrest would mean that candidates would be universally strong at this station, this has not proved to be the case and thorough practice of routines is the essential preparation for success.

Simulation

Simulators are now an established and validated part of the OSCE. In addition to the use of a simulator, as part of one resuscitation station as described above, a separate station uses an interactive simulator to create clinical problem scenarios. Although candidates may have no experience of this or any model of simulator, the monitoring displays are no different from those encountered in the anaesthetic room or operating theatre in real life and candidates should simply conduct themselves as they would if faced with the same problem in clinical practice. It is vitally important that candidates carefully read the information outside the station and also pay close attention to any changes in the clinical condition of the 'patient'. Correct laterality of the problem i.e. identification of the correct side, is a common source of error in these stimulated scenarios as is the tendency for candidates to assume a specific diagnosis and miss vital clues to the real problem.

Technical skills

Stations in this section test practical anaesthetic skills and the background knowledge associated with them. These can involve the use of mannequins and actors or volunteers. Whether a procedure needs to be carried out or simply demonstrated and explained will be made clear by the examiner, though obviously, if a human subject is being used, no insertion of needles or other equipment will be required.

Some skills tested may not be used frequently in everyday practice but are essential in managing uncommon but life-threatening situations. Knowledge of the equipment used for the procedures will be tested and marks for the safety aspects of procedures are generally weighted heavily. Anatomical knowledge may also be tested in some of the technical skill stations e.g. those related to regional anaesthetic techniques or invasive monitoring.

Example questions

These questions have been drawn from the existing bank of OSCE stations; some are in use, some are 'retired'. They provide a clear insight into the depth and scope of the individual stations. The questions are illustrative and should be of help to candidates in their preparations, and to tutors and others in devising practice stations for local use. Tutors and those setting up practice OSCEs will need to provide their own photographs and diagrams when creating stations; it has not been possible to include them in this book. A common theme is that they have clinical relevance and all of the questions relate to good, safe clinical practice.

Dr Campbell Edmondson, Chairman – OSCE Working Party

STRUCTURED ORAL EXAMINATION

The structured oral examination is designed to test understanding. Clearly, candidates still require a sound knowledge of the curriculum but questions are constructed to allow the examiners to probe deeper into this knowledge to assess the candidate's understanding of scientific principles and their application to clinical practice.

The SOE is in two parts, SOE 1 and SOE 2. Each part consists of six questions. SOE 1 starts with three questions in pharmacology followed by three in physiology while SOE 2 will start with three questions in clinical practice followed by three in physics. Each question lasts five minutes so each SOE part will last 30 minutes.

On entering the exam hall you should go straight to the cubicle identified by the letter allocated to you. You should enter and sit down. You will be greeted by two examiners who will conduct the exam for you. There may be another person sitting in the cubicle. This person is either a visitor or another examiner conducting an audit of the process. Neither will be involved in asking questions or marking your performance. Examiners only know candidates by their number and not name. As a result, it is possible that you may know the examiner in your allocated cubicle. If this is the case you should make this known to the floor supervisors who will move you to an adjacent cubicle.

When the bell sounds, the first examiner will ask you their set of three questions. Each question will last 5 minutes, resulting in the first half of the exam part which takes 15 minute. During this time the second examiner will write down details of the exchange. The bell will sound again and the two examiners will swap roles. After a further 15 minutes and three questions on the second section, the bell will sound again. This is then the end of this part of the exam and you may leave.

The two examiners will then mark your performance independently assessing each of the six topics as a fail (0 marks), borderline (1 mark) or pass (2 marks). The total scores of all four examiners are aggregated. A score of 37 or more out of 48 is needed to pass.

STRUCTURED ORAL EXAMINATION 1
PHYSIOLOGY AND PHARMACOLOGY

Structured Oral Examination part 1 (SOE 1) forms 50% of the total SOE mark and is examined in the morning. It is a test of understanding of the principles of pharmacology and physiology underlying anaesthesia, pain medicine and intensive care practice. The examination is 30 minutes long and consists of two sections of equal duration: 15 minutes of pharmacology followed by 15 minutes of physiology. During these 15 minutes, three topics are normally examined for approximately five minutes each. The examination is standardised for each candidate and always starts with 15 minutes of pharmacology. A standard opening question is used and the examiners will use a variety of questions following that to explore understanding and knowledge. These following questions may vary slightly between candidates in order to display their knowledge to the best of their ability.

The pharmacology and physiology SOE questions are all cross-referenced to the Basic Level Training curriculum. The questions are constantly reviewed and are changed to reflect changes in clinical practice and new developments in pharmacology and physiology. The performance of each question with regards to difficulty is known and each set of three questions are matched to ensure that each paper is of equal difficulty.

As with all parts of the SOE exam, the questions are used for two cohorts of candidates and then the questions are changed.

It is extremely important that you practise your SOE technique, as it is easy to think you know something and then fall short when you try to explain it. Ask senior colleagues and your peers to question you and give you feedback, the more you are used to verbalising explanations the easier it will be on the day.

For the pharmacology SOE, the three questions are taken from three broad areas of the syllabus. These three areas are anaesthetic pharmacology, the principles of pharmacology and general pharmacology. Anaesthetic pharmacology includes inhalational and intravenous agents, analgesic drugs, neuromuscular blocking agents and local anaesthetics. The principles of pharmacology questions may include aspects of drug handling by the body, including how drugs enter the body, their carriage and distribution, metabolism and excretion. Pharmacogenetics and statistics may also be examined. The general pharmacology question might explore a group of drugs such as B blockers; drugs used to treat a particular condition, such as oral hypoglycaemics, or a specific drug, such as a commonly prescribed antibiotic. To successfully answer a question it is important to demonstrate an understanding of pharmacological principles as well as being able to reproduce facts. If there are NICE guidelines regarding treatment of a given condition, such as Diabetes Mellitus, you should be aware of these. There are questions that ask you to compare the properties of a group of drugs, for instance inhalational anaesthetics, being able to rapidly provide the important properties of these drugs in tabular form will help you perform well in such questions.

Each question is given equal weighting in the marking system. The order that the questions are asked is always the same, anaesthetic, principles of pharmacology and general pharmacology.

The examination is constantly evolving, as our clinical practice evolves. There are questions that are relevant to intensive care medicine and pain medicine, as these are an important area of basic anaesthetic training.

In the physiology SOE, there will be an emphasis on cardiorespiratory physiology, which underpins our clinical practice. The following guide should help you understand how the oral examination is structured:

- The first question usually covers basic physiological topics such as cardiorespiratory, cell physiology or biochemistry.
- The second question is sometimes perceived as being more difficult by candidates as it will test knowledge of many of the body's control systems. This includes renal, endocrine and gastrointestinal, but other topics from the curriculum may also be tested.
- The third question may include important areas such as nerve and muscle physiology or body fluids, but may also include cardiorespiratory, if not previously tested.

It is important to have sound factual knowledge but unless you understand how to apply the knowledge, then it will be difficult to maximise your marks. There will be a number of questions which explore the inter relationships between the body systems and control mechanisms. These will normally relate to physiological changes caused by stresses to the body, for example: trauma, exercise and exposure to environmental variations. Changes caused by disease processes, such as pathophysiology, are more likely to be covered in the final exam.

The examiner may give you a graph with pre-drawn axes or a basic diagram which you will be asked to label to explain a physiological principle. Use these aids wherever possible, as it will give you more time to answer the questions.

Finally, be smart and professional. The SOE is a demanding examination but it can be very rewarding, so try your best to enjoy it. It is your chance to shine and express the knowledge and understanding that you have worked so hard to obtain. Good luck!

Dr Mark Forrest – Chair Pharmacology Group
Dr Tina McLeod – Chair Physiology Group

STRUCTURED ORAL EXAMINATION 2

Clinical Anaesthesia, Physics, Clinical Measurement, Equipment and Safety

The first half of SOE 2 always consists of the clinical anaesthesia questions. In the ten minutes prior to entering the examinations room, candidates will be given a laminated sheet containing a short description of a clinical case scenario. There may possibly be some additional clinical material, such as blood results or an ECG, on the sheet. To avoid having to commit details to memory, an identical sheet will be on the table in front of the candidates when they are being examined. The cases are chosen so as to be suitable for anaesthetists in their second year of training, and the standard of questioning will be aimed at this level. They will thus not include very detailed cases from sub-specialties of anaesthesia, such as neurosurgery, cardiac or neonatal anaesthesia and all questions will only cover areas that are included within the curriculum. Cases may, however, include some situations where an on-call anaesthetic CT2 may have to initiate management whilst awaiting senior help, for example, resuscitation of an unconscious, critically ill patient in the emergency department or the care of an injured 8 year old following an accident.

The 15 minute clinical part of the SOE is divided into three approximately equal parts of five minutes. This allows for several areas of the case to be explored. These might include:

- relevant aspects of the history and/or associated medical problems
- aspects of the anaesthetic management of the case, usually involving a form of problem solving scenario or critical incident
- topics related to the further management of this case, perhaps post-operatively, including options for suitable post-operative analgesia.

Candidates must, of course, be able to demonstrate adequate factual knowledge, but it is also important to show a logical and systematic approach to dealing with common topics, such as medical co-morbidities and critical incidents. If candidates do not appear to be able to deal with common problems, this will be reflected in the final mark. We would also expect candidates to show a mature approach to calling for senior help. In situations where it is appropriate to call for help, we would expect candidates to do so. However, that is not an end in itself, and candidates should still be able to demonstrate that they are clinically capable and decisive. A candidate will need to describe how they would institute appropriate treatment whilst help is on its way.

After 15 minutes have elapsed, the half-time bell will sound. At this point, the examiners will swap over. The second examiner will ask the questions in the remaining section of the SOE, while the first one now records the topics covered.

There are three question topics of approximately five minutes each, chosen in no particular order from the Clinical Measurement, Physics, Equipment and Safety Curriculum. The same three questions are asked in the same order at each examiner's table.

The questions are set well before the examination. We know how easy or difficult candidates have found each question in the past and so we are able, as far as possible, to make sure no paper is significantly more difficult than another.

Anything that is in the curriculum may be asked. It is therefore very unwise not to revise a particular topic in the hope that 'it may not come up'. Subjects may be repeated later in the week, so knowledge of previously asked questions is of no assistance in predicting later topics.

In both sections of the SOE, the examiners will have been given an opening question with which to start the examination. This means that candidates all get the same opportunity to answer without being put off by a poorly phrased or convoluted question at the start. In the Physics section, the opening question may sometimes be worded so as to illustrate that the subject matter is relevant to clinical anaesthesia. The questions may then develop along different lines, although there is a list of areas within each topic that the examiner has to cover during the five minutes. It is this that gives the structure to the examination, ensuring questions asked are only from the curriculum and are similar for each candidate.

It is important that candidates are tested on the same key topics but that examiners have the opportunity to explore each candidate's depth of understanding before moving on. Examiners thus respond to the answers of the candidate to test understanding before moving on. Questions are used for two successive cohorts of candidates before being changed.

In both sections of the SOE, it is possible that the examiners will use supporting material. Diagrams, photographs or graphs may be used at the start of questioning or introduced later on.

Candidates may be asked to draw a simple diagram themselves if they think it would help their explanation. Paper and pencils are provided at the tables for this.

However:

- diagrams are not compulsory
- diagrams can be used to help demonstrate your understanding of a topic if used wisely
- diagrams should be large, clear and relevant
- detailed works of art are not required – there are no marks for artistic merit
- use the time whilst drawing; do not waste time, explain what you are doing as you go along
- do not attempt to draw a diagram if you are uncertain of your facts
- label graphs, use appropriate units, draw the right shaped line in the right place
- beware applying excessive force to the disposable propelling pencils, causing the lead to break!

After the final bell has gone and candidates have left the room, the examiners will award marks independently.

It is not possible to ignore whole sections of the syllabus in the hope that good performance elsewhere will pull up the overall mark and result in a pass. Significant gaps in knowledge and understanding will almost certainly result in a low overall mark and failure of the SOE component of the Primary exam.

Examiners try hard to make the exam as fair as possible and try to get the best out of every candidate. We much prefer to celebrate success than commiserate with failure!

Dr Cleave Gass – Chair Clinical Group
Dr Chris Leng – Chair Physics Group

Results, guidance, review, appeal and complaint procedures

A guidance interview for unsuccessful examination candidates has been an integral part of the College's approach to examination failure since November 1990. With the changes to the delivery and marking of the examination in the past three years, candidates have routinely been provided with an increased amount of information in respect of their performance in the various components of the exam. Currently, pass or fail results for the MCQ are placed on the website on a specified date and followed up by a formal letter, which provides the pass mark, the candidate's score for the overall exam and the score for each subsection. Pass or Fail results for the OSCE, SOE and Primary exam overall are normally placed on the website from 2pm on the following working day. This is followed up by formal letter, which provides the pass marks for each component, the candidate's total scores for the OSCE and SOE, plus the scores for each OSCE station and SOE subsection, examiner's comments at the SOE are also available on request.

The provision of this information, coupled with the ability of a candidate to retain a pass in a component of the examination, led to a re-evaluation of the need and the purpose of guidance. In September 2010, the College decided that there was no longer a mandatory requirement for a candidate to attend examination guidance interviews except at the sixth and final attempt. Any candidate who repeatedly fails a component of the exam may, however, request for an interview with an FRCA examiner in regard to addressing shortfalls in examination performance.

Interviews are limited to one per examination part, i.e. Primary OSCE and/or SOE, Final Written and Final SOE. Guidance is not offered for the Primary MCQ. Requests should be made by email (exams@rcoa.ac.uk) from the College Tutor, or senior consultant for non-trainees, to the examinations department, within one calendar month of the date of the last failed exam component. Where such interviews are approved, the attendance of a College Tutor is strongly encouraged.

No special consideration is given in respect of refunds following guidance interviews. Non request of a guidance only affects eligibility towards examinations at the sixth attempt.

Examination guidance interviews last 20/30 minutes and are undertaken by one or more experienced examiners; this may include a Primary and/or Final examiner. The atmosphere is informal and the interviewee is advised that, despite the appearance of an examination oral format, the object of the exercise is to identify weaknesses in examination performance and to offer constructive guidance on how to better prepare for the next attempt. Before the interview, the candidate is asked to complete a form, which has a section for input by the College Tutor or a local mentor, and which provides useful background information to the interview. On request, interviews are offered as soon as possible, following the exam sitting. Wherever possible interviews will be held regionally. This will hopefully allow more College Tutors/mentors to accompany their candidates, so that the best possible plan of interactive preparation for the next examination can be discussed.

After the interview, a synopsis of examination performance and the advice given is sent to the candidate and, with the candidate's permission, to the College Tutor.

In situations where a candidate feels aggrieved by the examinations process they have the right to request a review of the conduct or the result of their examination. Reviews will be entertained which allege impropriety or bias of some kind in the organisation, content, conduct or determination of the result of the examination. No review, however, may be made of matters which relate solely to the examiners' judgment. If, on completion of a review decision a candidate remains dissatisfied, he/she may submit a request for an appeal, which must be applied for using the application form at Annex A of the College Examination Regulations (Reviews and Appeals) and accompanied by the appropriate fee. Full details can be found on the College website www.rcoa.ac.uk/examinations/overview/regulations.

The College recognises that on occasions candidates may wish to express their dissatisfaction with the way in which something has been done and feel confident that any such complaint is handled in a fair and consistent way. Candidates who consider that they have grounds for complaint, regarding the provision of a service by the College that does not amount to a request for a 'review' should use the regulations set out in the Examination Regulations (Reviews and Appeals) at paragraphs 20-30. All complaints should be brought to the attention of a College office as soon as possible so that immediate action can be taken to resolve issues wherever possible.

Dr Mike Wilkinson/Dr Jane Bembridge

QUESTIONS

2

MCQ examination

The following 90 questions have been selected in the same way as an actual paper. The layout is exactly as it would be in the examination. There are 60 Multiple True False (MTF) questions in three subsections: 20 pharmacology, 20 physiology and 20 physics (including clinical measurement and statistics). There then follow 30 Single Best Answer (SBA) questions in the same categories, although some clinical questions may test knowledge and its application in more than one category. Questions on applied clinical anatomy are included in the physiology subsection.

Dr Anthony McCluskey

MTF Questions 1–20: Pharmacology

1 Cisatracurium:

-] **a** is one of two stereoisomers in atracurium
-] **b** is of equal potency to atracurium
-] **c** undergoes direct hydrolysis by plasma esterases
-] **d** has no active metabolites
-] **e** is more dependent than atracurium on renal function for excretion

2 Propofol:

-] **a** is a water soluble phenol compound
-] **b** has an elimination half-life of less than one hour
-] **c** glucuronidation occurs through the hydroxyl group at position 1
-] **d** acts only on the β subunit of the GABA receptor
-] **e** has anti-emetic effects which may be due to dopamine antagonism

3 The following are true of local anaesthetic drugs:

-] **a** lidocaine and tetracaine (amethocaine) are both amides
-] **b** potency is related to lipid solubility
-] **c** rate of onset of action is independent of dose administered
-] **d** ropivacaine is more potent than lidocaine
-] **e** ester local anaesthetic drugs are all poorly bound to plasma proteins

4 Phase I depolarisation blockade:

-] **a** shows 'fade' during tetanic stimulation
-] **b** may be potentiated by anticholinesterases
-] **c** shows post-tetanic facilitation
-] **d** is prolonged by prior administration of a small dose of a non-depolarising relaxant
-] **e** is antagonised by dantrolene

5 Adverse effects of heparin include:

- **a** thrombocytopenia
- **b** hyperkalaemia
- **c** hypersensitivity reactions
- **d** intra-uterine fetal haemorrhage
- **e** osteoporosis

6 The rapid intravenous administration of 2 grams of mannitol per kilogram of body weight will induce:

- **a** a decrease in serum sodium
- **b** low osmolality of the plasma
- **c** hypervolaemia
- **d** a decrease in intracellular osmolality
- **e** reduction in the volume of the brain

7 The following are true of diuretics:

- **a** large doses of mannitol increase extracellular osmolarity
- **b** acetazolamide decreases urinary pH
- **c** thiazide drugs inhibit sodium reabsorption in the distal tubule
- **d** furosemide decreases the ototoxicity of aminoglycoside antibiotics
- **e** bumetanide inhibits electrolyte reabsorption in the ascending Loop of Henle

8 The following drugs may potentiate warfarin:

- **a** rifampicin
- **b** aspirin
- **c** paracetamol
- **d** amiodarone
- **e** tamoxifen

9 Ketamine:

- **a** is an antagonist at glutamate receptors
- **b** is a butyrophenone derivative
- **c** is presented as a racemic mixture
- **d** causes bronchodilatation
- **e** has a direct positive inotropic effect

10 The following statements regarding intravenous induction agents are correct:

- **a** etomidate is approximately 2.5 times more potent than thiopental
- **b** ketamine is metabolised in the liver
- **c** propofol emulsion has a pH of 7
- **d** thiopental has a high hepatic extraction ratio
- **e** etomidate is broken down by ester hydrolysis

11 The following statements concerning benzodiazepines are correct:

- **a** they act at $GABA_A$ and $GABA_B$ receptors
- **b** lorazepam has active metabolites
- **c** they can cause ataxia and impaired motor co-ordination
- **d** they cause a decrease in plasma chloride concentration
- **e** midazolam can be administered by the rectal and intranasal routes

12 True statements about bronchodilating agents include:

- **a** salmeterol has a longer duration of action but a slower onset and should not be used to treat acute asthmatic attacks
- **b** isoproterenol (isoprenaline) has both beta-1 and beta-2 adrenergic actions
- **c** aminophylline increases cyclic AMP through inhibition of phosphodiesterase
- **d** salbutamol increases the activity of adenylyl cyclase
- **e** salbutamol lowers serum potassium concentration

13 Alfentanil:

- a is 90% unionised at pH 7.4
- b has a higher clearance than morphine
- c has a smaller volume of distribution than fentanyl
- d is more potent than fentanyl
- e is more protein bound than pethidine

14 Cyclizine:

- a has a duration of effect of one hour
- b is a potent inhibitor of gastric acid secretion
- c 80% is excreted unchanged by the kidney
- d has an atropine-like effect
- e is non-sedating

15 The following are true of non-steroidal anti-inflammatory drugs (NSAIDs):

- a NSAIDs are highly bound to albumin in the plasma
- b NSAIDs have a volume of distribution greater than 500 ml kg^{-1}
- c parenteral administration of NSAIDs ensures that gastric mucosal damage does not occur
- d it is safe to use COX-2 inhibitors in the presence of established ischaemic heart disease
- e NSAIDs enhance platelet aggregation

16 Sevoflurane:

- a has a boiling point of 48°C
- b has a saturated vapour pressure at 20°C of 21 kPa (160 mm Hg)
- c is metabolised to a greater extent than desflurane
- d is a respiratory stimulant at low concentrations
- e relaxes bronchial smooth muscle

17 The MAC value of an inhalational anaesthetic agent may be decreased by:

- **a** clonidine
- **b** neostigmine
- **c** amphetamine
- **d** methyldopa
- **e** digoxin

18 Drugs whose action is prolonged in patients with acute renal failure include:

- **a** morphine
- **b** ranitidine
- **c** alfentanil
- **d** propofol
- **e** labetalol

19 Diamorphine:

- **a** is a naturally occurring opioid
- **b** is more lipid soluble than morphine
- **c** has a higher affinity for opioid receptors than morphine
- **d** is well absorbed after subcutaneous administration
- **e** is converted to monoacetylmorphine

20 Hypoglycaemic agents with a rapid onset of action (less than one hour) include:

- **a** soluble insulin
- **b** insulin glargine
- **c** insulin lispro
- **d** protamine zinc insulin
- **e** isophane insulin

21 The anterior lobe of the pituitary gland:

- **a** synthesises vasopressin
- **b** has important neural connections with the pineal body
- **c** develops separately from the posterior lobe
- **d** contains chromophobe cells
- **e** has a portal blood supply independent of the posterior lobe

22 The glomerular filtrate normally contains:

- **a** inulin in a lower concentration than in plasma when given to measure glomerular filtration rate
- **b** albumin at 5% of its plasma concentration
- **c** amino acids
- **d** glucose in a concentration equal to that in plasma
- **e** no uric acid

23 The metabolic response to injury includes:

- **a** catabolism
- **b** retention of potassium in the body
- **c** hypoglycaemia
- **d** raised plasma cortisol concentration
- **e** increased production of epinephrine

24 Pulmonary variables that decrease during pregnancy include:

- **a** minute ventilation
- **b** PaO_2
- **c** $PaCO_2$
- **d** FRC
- **e** total respiratory compliance

25 The cell-mediated immune response:

- **a** provides an explanation for some auto-immune diseases
- **b** involves peripheral sensitisation of lymphocytes
- **c** causes proliferation of plasma cells
- **d** involves increased IgM synthesis
- **e** causes massive release of histamine

26 Ptosis results from damage to the:

- **a** oculomotor nerve
- **b** parasympathetic supply of the eye
- **c** cervical sympathetic chain
- **d** trigeminal nerve
- **e** supra-orbital nerve

27 In the cerebrospinal fluid of a normal individual:

- **a** the reduced buffering capacity is mainly due to a lower bicarbonate concentration
- **b** pH is the same as that of arterial blood
- **c** protein concentration is less than in plasma
- **d** chloride concentration is higher than in venous blood
- **e** glucose concentration is higher than in arterial blood

28 In the liver:

- **a** hepatic arterial blood flow exceeds portal blood flow
- **b** the bile canaliculus is at the centre of the lobule
- **c** the portal vein contributes approximately one third of the total hepatic blood flow
- **d** portal venous pressure normally exceeds 20 mm Hg
- **e** the oxygen tension is lowest at the centre of the lobule

29 Consequences of 24 hours starvation include:

] **a** increased brain uptake of glucose

] **b** reduction of the respiratory quotient

] **c** elevated blood glucagon concentration

] **d** increased urinary nitrogen output

] **e** development of metabolic alkalosis

30 The following are examples of active transport of substances across membranes:

] **a** movement of sodium out of a nerve

] **b** reabsorption of water in the proximal renal tubule

] **c** movement of water across the collecting duct

] **d** iodide uptake by the thyroid gland

] **e** hydrogen ion secretion by the gastric parietal cells

31 Albumin:

] **a** is absorbed from the large bowel

] **b** is filtered at the glomeruli in significant quantities

] **c** is a specific carrier protein

] **d** has antibody properties

] **e** has a molecular weight of approximately 70,000 daltons

32 Closing volume:

] **a** is greater than closing capacity

] **b** is attributed to collapse of segmental bronchi in dependent parts of the lung

] **c** tends to increase with age

] **d** is measured by the helium dilution technique

] **e** is reduced by moving from the supine to the upright position

33 The oxyhaemoglobin dissociation curve:

- **a** may be used to calculate the P_{50}
- **b** indicates the oxygen carrying capacity of the blood
- **c** is displaced to the left in anaemia
- **d** has the same shape as the carboxyhaemoglobin dissociation curve
- **e** is displaced to the left by passive hyperventilation

34 Airway resistance:

- **a** can be measured using a body plethysmograph
- **b** is expressed as litres kPa^{-1}
- **c** is independent of lung volume
- **d** is increased in forced expiration
- **e** is independent of flow

35 A subject acutely exposed to an inspired oxygen concentration of 10% at sea level will:

- **a** develop respiratory alkalosis
- **b** secrete a more acid urine
- **c** have increased pulmonary vasoconstriction
- **d** have an increased cardiac output
- **e** respond immediately by increasing erythropoietin production

36 Important determinants of myocardial oxygen consumption include:

- **a** heart rate
- **b** ventricular wall tension
- **c** myocardial contractility
- **d** left ventricular end-diastolic volume
- **e** pulmonary capillary wedge pressure

37 Blood vessels that contribute to physiological shunt include the:

- **a** coronary sinus
- **b** Thebesian veins
- **c** anterior cardiac vein
- **d** bronchial venous drainage
- **e** ductus venosus

38 Intracranial pressure:

- **a** is decreased by hypoxia
- **b** can be reduced by hyperventilation
- **c** is lower when intra-thoracic pressure is low
- **d** rises following head injury and should be treated with systemic steroids
- **e** may be estimated by the Kety-Schmidt method

39 Urinary osmolality increases in response to:

- **a** aldosterone
- **b** vasopressin
- **c** cortisol
- **d** dehydration
- **e** increased dietary protein

40 The tendon jerks in the lower limb are reduced if, fifty days previously, the:

- **a** lumbo-sacral anterior horn cells are damaged
- **b** ipsilateral pyramidal tract is interrupted in the spinal cord
- **c** contralateral internal capsule is damaged
- **d** motor cortex is damaged on the contralateral side
- **e** ipsilateral spino-thalamic tract is interrupted by disease

MTF Questions 41–60: Physics, Clinical Measurement and Statistics

41 When measuring central venous pressure:

- a a catheter inserted in an adult at the antecubital fossa should be passed no more than 20 cm up the vein
- b the optimum internal diameter for the catheter is 0.25 mm
- c direct subclavian vein catheterisation can be used
- d microshock is a potential hazard
- e the zero level should be set at the level of the angle of Louis whatever the position of the patient

42 A liquid inhalational anaesthetic agent is allowed to come into equilibrium with a mixture of gases. Under these conditions, the partial pressure of the agent in the resulting gas mixture depends on:

- a the atmospheric pressure
- b the surface area of the liquid
- c the volume of the liquid
- d the temperature of the liquid
- e the composition of the gas mixture

43 The correct SI unit for:

- a force is the pascal
- b mass is the gram
- c time is the second
- d length is the metre
- e energy is the watt

44 The following are true of critical temperature:

] **a** critical temperature is the temperature above which a substance cannot be liquefied however much pressure is applied

] **b** the critical temperature of oxygen is -119°C

] **c** nitrous oxide cylinders always contain liquid nitrous oxide

] **d** the critical temperature of nitrous oxide is 48.5°C

] **e** critical pressure is the vapour pressure of a substance at its critical temperature

45 According to laws of physics:

] **a** Boyle's Law assumes that molecular size is unimportant

] **b** Boyle's Law states that the volume of a gas varies inversely with pressure

] **c** Charles' Law predicts that as the temperature of a mass of gas is raised from 10°C to 20°C its volume will double

] **d** Dalton's Law states that a gas dissolves in proportion to its partial pressure

] **e** Laplace's Law suggests that large alveoli should collapse

46 The Doppler effect:

] **a** applies to both electromagnetic radiation and sound

] **b** changes the velocity of reflected ultrasound

] **c** depends on the piezo-electric properties of some crystals

] **d** shows a shift to lower frequency if the source is moving away from the receiver

] **e** can indicate the velocity of red blood cells

47 Sevoflurane vapour:

] **a** concentration can be measured using a refractometer

] **b** is less dense than air

] **c** absorbs ultraviolet radiation

] **d** can be measured by absorption of infrared radiation

] **e** can be measured by mass spectrometry

48 The Bain coaxial breathing system:

] **a** delivers the fresh gas flow in the outer tube

] **b** requires a fresh gas flow equal to the patient's minute volume to prevent rebreathing with spontaneous respiration

] **c** can be used in a child weighing 20 kg

] **d** has a dead space which is increased if the inner tube is dislodged at the machine end

] **e** can function as a Mapleson C system

49 The following are true of piped gases:

] **a** the normal pipeline pressure for nitrous oxide is 4.1 Bar

] **b** the changeover valve incorporated in a cylinder bank works on a pneumatic shuttle mechanism

] **c** the non-interchangeability of Schrader valves depends on varying sizes of collars on the probes

] **d** the Schrader outlet contains an internal non-return valve

] **e** when reinstating oxygen pipelines after servicing, testing with an oxygen analyser ensures the integrity of the system

50 The following are true of the measurement of oxygen concentration:

] **a** oxygen is a paramagnetic gas because its molecule has paired electrons in the outer shell

] **b** in a paramagnetic analyser, the two glass spheres are filled with oxygen

] **c** in a paramagnetic analyser, rotation of the dumb-bell is balanced by torsion in a suspending filament

] **d** in a null-deflection analyser, an opposing magnetic field prevents movement of the dumb-bell

] **e** water vapour affects paramagnetic oxygen analysis

51 The following are true of viscosity:

- a established turbulent flow is independent of viscosity
- b viscosity of blood increases with plasma protein concentration
- c increased viscosity reduces blood flow
- d low temperature raises blood viscosity
- e helium improves gas flow through an orifice by reducing viscosity

52 The following are true of manometers:

- a 7.5 mm mercury is equivalent to 10.2 cm water
- b 1 kPa is equal to a pressure of 7.5 mm mercury
- c the top of a mercury manometer is closed to prevent contamination and spillage
- d a mercury barometer used to measure atmospheric pressure is sealed with a vacuum above the surface of the liquid
- e aneroid gauges do not contain liquid

53 Measurement of peak expiratory flow rate:

- a reveals a normal diurnal variation of less than 10%
- b is made ideally using a Vitalograph
- c with a Wright's peak flow meter uses the principle of a constant orifice with a variable pressure drop
- d can be achieved using a 'rapid' capnograph
- e produces a reading which is normally 450 - 650 L min^{-1} in the adult

54 Transducers:

- a convert one form of energy into another
- b amplify the original signal
- c can be active or passive
- d display a physiological event on an oscilloscope
- e are used in the measurement of body temperature

55 The following are true of the measurement of body fluid volumes:

- **a** total blood volume can be measured directly using inulin
- **b** extracellular fluid volume is measured using deuterium oxide or tritium
- **c** intracellular fluid volume is measured indirectly from extracellular volume and total body water
- **d** plasma volume is measured with radio-iodinated albumin
- **e** total red cell volume is measured with chromium-labelled red cells

56 Anaesthetic gas cylinders:

- **a** are made of galvanised steel
- **b** for nitrous oxide contain it as a liquid
- **c** filling ratio is the volume of the cylinder contents divided by the volume of water the cylinder could hold
- **d** filling ratio for nitrous oxide in the UK is 0.9
- **e** may cool if gas flow rates are high

57 In a well designed clinical study:

- **a** a power of 50% is satisfactory
- **b** double blinding ensures only the investigators are aware of the nature of the treatment
- **c** a pilot study can predict the number of patients required
- **d** confidence intervals in each group are large
- **e** a Chi Squared test can compare the sex distribution

58 The standard deviation of a sample from a normally distributed characteristic in a population:

- **a** describes the degree of bias in choosing the sample
- **b** determines the deviation about the mean which half the values might be expected to show
- **c** is the square root of the variance
- **d** identifies limits of the deviation either side of the mean which include approximately two-thirds of the values
- **e** is greater than the standard error of the mean

59 For the eight observations: 0,1,1,1,2,4,5,10:

- **a** the range is 1 to 10
- **b** the standard deviation is a good measure of dispersion
- **c** the median is 1.5
- **d** the distribution is skewed
- **e** the distribution is bimodal

60 The following are true of electrical safety:

- **a** skin impedance is increased if faulty apparatus is touched with wet hands
- **b** electrical shock is not a risk with potentials below 24V AC or 50V DC
- **c** the modern diathermy return plate is not connected directly to earth
- **d** microshock can cause ventricular fibrillation via an intracardiac catheter with current of 150 microamps
- **e** leakage currents are caused by voltages induced in other circuits by alternating mains current

Questions 61–90: Single Best Answer Questions

61 A 56 year-old man with a one hour history of chest pain presents to the Emergency Department. Blood pressure is 70/45 mm Hg, heart rate 115 min^{-1} and regular to palpation. On examination he is cyanosed and his peripheries are cold and clammy. A 12-lead ECG has not yet been performed.

The most important <u>immediate</u> treatment for this patient is:

- **a** Clopidogrel
- **b** Fibrinolytic therapy
- **c** Glyceryl trinitrate
- **d** High flow oxygen
- **e** Nifedipine

62 A ventilated patient has been admitted to the Intensive Care Unit after emergency major colorectal surgery and is receiving a continuous intravenous infusion of a drug to support his cardiovascular system. Blood glucose concentration 12 h later is 13 mmol L^{-1} although he is not known to be diabetic. You suspect that the choice of drug infusion may be responsible.

The drug infusion is most likely to be which of the following?

- **a** Adrenaline
- **b** Dobutamine
- **c** Enoximone
- **d** Noradrenaline
- **e** Vasopressin

63 **A patient undergoes removal of sebaceous cyst under total intravenous general anaesthesia using propofol and alfentanil. The surgeon infiltrates local anaesthetic at the end of surgery.**

Which of the following properties of alfentanil is the best reason for choosing it rather than fentanyl?

- **a** Clearance
- **b** Inactive metabolites
- **c** pKa
- **d** Potency
- **e** Volume of distribution

64 **An asthmatic develops severe bronchospasm after administration of diclofenac.**

This is most likely to be caused by production of:

- **a** Arachidonic acid
- **b** Leukotrienes
- **c** Phospholipase A2
- **d** Prostacyclin
- **e** Thromboxane A2

65 **A 12.5 kg two-year-old boy requires hernia repair as a day case. After induction of general anaesthesia a caudal block is performed using levobupivacaine for intra-operative and post-operative analgesia.**

Which of the following doses is most appropriate?

- **a** 0.25%, 10 ml
- **b** 0.25%, 20 ml
- **c** 0.5%, 5 ml
- **d** 0.5%, 10 ml
- **e** 0.75%, 3 ml

66 A patient with chronic renal failure receiving an intravenous diamorphine infusion has had a respiratory arrest.

Which of the following is the most likely cause?

- **a** Decreased plasma clearance of diamorphine
- **b** Decreased plasma volume following dialysis leading to increased plasma concentration of diamorphine
- **c** Impaired renal excretion of diamorphine
- **d** Increased plasma concentration of 6-monoacetyl morphine
- **e** Increased plasma concentration of morphine-6-glucuronide

67 A new aminosteroid non-depolarising neuromuscular blocker with a similar molecular weight to rocuronium produces satisfactory intubating conditions 45 seconds after administration.

Which of the following is most likely to be a property of the new drug?

- **a** Clinical intubating dose 2 mg Kg^{-1}
- **b** Greater potency than rocuronium
- **c** Muscle fasciculation
- **d** Recovery of train-of-four ratio > 0.9 within 15 minutes
- **e** Reversed by sugammadex

68 An experiment is being designed to assess speed of gastric emptying. It is planned to administer a standard dose of a marker drug orally to healthy volunteers and then measure plasma drug concentrations at standard times after the oral dose.

Which of the following drugs is likely to be most useful in this experiment?

- **a** Aspirin
- **b** Morphine
- **c** Paracetamol
- **d** Propranolol
- **e** Vancomycin

69 A new phenylpiperidine opioid analgesic is found to have a potency ten times that of morphine. Its pKa is 6.1 and it is metabolised in the liver with a clearance of 10 ml Kg^{-1}. Its volume of distribution at steady state is 8 L Kg^{-1} and it is 75% plasma protein bound.

Which of the following properties of the new drug is the most likely explanation for it having a faster onset time than fentanyl?

- **a** Degree of plasma protein binding
- **b** Hepatic clearance
- **c** pKa
- **d** Potency
- **e** Volume of distribution

70 **A 72-year-old patient in the Acute Medical Admissions Unit has persistent bradycardia with a blood pressure of 110/50 mm Hg. He denies chest pain or shortness of breath but has experienced several episodes of dizziness. He is currently receiving 40% oxygen by facemask, his oxygen saturation is 96% and he looks comfortable. His ECG shows regular p-waves at a rate of 80 min^{-1} and regular QRS complexes of 0.16 ms duration at a rate of 30 min^{-1}.**

Which of the following is the most important <u>immediate</u> treatment?

- **a** Adrenaline
- **b** Atropine
- **c** Ephedrine
- **d** Glucagon
- **e** Pacing

71 **An intravenous infusion of a drug is administered to a 60 kg subject and, at steady state, urine is collected over four hours from a urinary catheter. The following data are obtained:**

Plasma concentration at steady state = 25 mcg ml^{-1}

Urinary concentration = 2.5 mg ml^{-1}

Total urlnary volume = 240 ml

What is the renal clearance of the substance?

- **a** 24 ml min^{-1}
- **b** 60 ml min^{-1}
- **c** 100 ml min^{-1}
- **d** 120 ml min^{-1}
- **e** 240 ml min^{-1}

72 **Myocardial contractility may be defined as the intrinsic ability of cardiac muscle fibres to do work with a given preload and afterload.**

Which of the following is the best measure of left ventricular (LV) contractility?

- **a** Ejection fraction
- **b** LV end-diastolic pressure
- **c** LV end-diastolic volume
- **d** LV end-systolic pressure
- **e** Stroke volume

73 **A patient with a history of ischaemic heart disease is complaining of central chest pain following laparoscopic cholecystectomy. A 12-lead ECG shows ST elevation in leads II, III and aVF.**

Which coronary artery is most likely to have been occluded?

- **a** Left anterior descending artery
- **b** Left circumflex artery
- **c** Left coronary artery
- **d** Posterior interventricular artery
- **e** Right coronary artery

74 Oxygen delivery to skeletal muscle may increase by a factor of 50 during vigorous exercise.

Which of the following physiological changes increases oxygen delivery to skeletal muscle during exercise by the greatest multiple?

- **a** Decreased parasympathetic tone to skeletal muscle
- **b** Increased cardiac output
- **c** Increased partial pressure gradient for oxygen between capillary blood and mitochondria
- **d** Relaxation of skeletal muscle precapillary sphincters
- **e** Right shift of the haemoglobin-oxygen dissociation curve

75 The pH of venous blood is only slightly lower than that of arterial blood despite the addition of large amounts of CO_2 in the tissues.

Which of the following is the best explanation for this?

- **a** Bohr effect
- **b** Buffering of H^+ ions by plasma proteins
- **c** Carbon dioxide is very soluble in blood
- **d** Carbonic anhydrase activity
- **e** Haldane effect

76 A patient with a body mass index of 50 Kg m^{-2} and no other medical history of note is scheduled for surgery under general anaesthesia. The ODP has changed his position from semi-sitting to horizontal for induction of anaesthesia.

Which of the following is the most important respiratory change that will occur?

- **a** Chest compliance will decrease
- **b** Functional residual capacity will decrease
- **c** Inspiratory reserve volume will increase
- **d** Peak expiratory flow rate will decrease
- **e** Respiratory rate will increase

77 Oxygen delivery to the tissues (oxygen flux) increases during normal pregnancy.

Which of the following is the most important reason for this?

- **a** Increased myocardial contractility
- **b** Increased haematocrit
- **c** Increased PaO_2
- **d** Increased venous return
- **e** Shift of the oxygen-haemoglobin dissociation curve

78 In an experimental situation, a giant squid axon is bathed in an electrolyte solution containing chloride, potassium and sodium ions.

Which of the following changes would have the greatest effect in making the resting membrane potential less negative?

- **a** Decreasing the extracellular concentration of potassium ions
- **b** Decreasing the extracellular concentration of sodium ions
- **c** Increasing the extracellular concentration of chloride ions
- **d** Increasing the extracellular concentration of potassium ions
- **e** Increasing the extracellular concentration of sodium ions

79 Systemic vascular resistance (SVR) can be calculated if cardiac output has been measured.

Which of the following additional pairs of measurements is needed to calculate SVR?

- **a** Diastolic and systolic systemic arterial pressure
- **b** Diastolic systemic arterial pressure and pulmonary artery occlusion pressure
- **c** Left ventricular end-diastolic pressure and mean systemic arterial pressure
- **d** Mean systemic arterial pressure and central venous pressure
- **e** Mean pulmonary artery pressure and central venous pressure

80 In order to investigate the factors determining the ventilatory response to hypercapnia, healthy volunteers breathe through a tight-fitting facemask connected to a breathing system containing 21% oxygen and 7% carbon dioxide.

Which of the following is the most important factor that directly drives the observed change in minute ventilation?

- **a** Increased hydrogen ion concentration of arterial blood
- **b** Increased hydrogen ion concentration of CSF
- **c** Stimulation of the carotid bodies
- **d** Stimulation of central chemoreceptors by increased $PaCO_2$
- **e** Stimulation of peripheral chemoreceptors by increased $PaCO_2$

81 A patient is receiving oxygen therapy using a Venturi face mask with an entrainment ratio of approximately 1:10 and oxygen flow rate of 6 L min^{-1}.

What is the approximate inspired oxygen concentration?

- **a** 24%
- **b** 28%
- **c** 35%
- **d** 40%
- **e** 60%

82 **An isoflurane vapouriser calibrated at sea level is being used at high altitude. The anaesthetist uses the vapouriser making no allowance for altitude. Maintenance of anaesthesia using a vapouriser setting of 1.0-1.5% isoflurane in air appears to run uneventfully.**

Which of the following best explains why the anaesthetist may use the same dial settings on the vapouriser at high altitude as at sea level?

- **a** Depth of anaesthesia is titrated against clinical response not anaesthetic concentration
- **b** Isoflurane concentration at the vapouriser output increases as ambient pressure decreases
- **c** Monitors of end-tidal vapour concentration compensate for altitude
- **d** Plenum vapourisers deliver the same partial pressure at any particular dial setting irrespective of ambient pressure
- **e** The temperature drop at higher altitudes has only minimal effect on vapouriser function

83 **Ultrasound (US) machines have various controls to alter the quality of the image seen on screen.**

Which of the following best explains how image quality is optimised when increasing the depth of focus from 2 cm to 6 cm?

- **a** More US waves are emitted from the probe
- **b** The wavelength of the US wave is increased
- **c** The image is enhanced by digital processing
- **d** The US transducer is recalibrated to be more sensitive
- **e** The US transducer output is amplified to a greater extent

84 An oxygen Rotameter bobbin reads a flow rate 1 L min^{-1}. As the Rotameter needle valve is opened further, the bobbin rises up the tube and then comes to rest at a reading of 8 L min^{-1}.

Which of the following descriptions of the physics of gas flow around the bobbin best explains why the bobbin comes to rest opposite the 8 L min^{-1} marker?

- **a** The cross sectional area of the Rotameter tube has increased
- **b** The flow has become less laminar
- **c** The flow has become more turbulent
- **d** The forces acting above and below the bobbin have equalised
- **e** The pressure gradient across the bobbin has remained constant during its ascent

85 Nitrous oxide cylinders have a Bourdon pressure gauge attached. A partially used cylinder contains nitrous oxide liquid and vapour.

Which of the following is the best explanation as to why the pressure gauge cannot be used to estimate the contents of this nitrous oxide cylinder, which is not currently in use?

- **a** The critical temperature of nitrous oxide is approximately 36.5°C
- **b** The cylinder contents can only be estimated by weighing the cylinder
- **c** The pressure gauge will indicate SVP at ambient temperature for nitrous oxide regardless of the cylinder contents
- **d** The pressure gauge reading falls when the cylinder is in use
- **e** The pressure gauge reading is temperature dependent

86 **A patient is ventilated using a circle system with a fresh gas flow (FGF) of 500 ml min^{-1}. The capnograph trace is of normal morphology with a plateau at 8.2 kPa and a baseline at 2.1 kPa.**

What is the single most important <u>immediate</u> course of action?

- **a** Check the patient's core temperature
- **b** Increase the fresh gas flow
- **c** Increase the FiO_2
- **d** Increase the minute ventilation
- **e** Replace the soda lime

87 **With patients routinely connected to a variety of electrical equipment in the operating theatre, safety is paramount.**

Which of the following is the most important electrical safety feature of such equipment?

- **a** A current-operated earth leakage circuit breaker is in place
- **b** An isolation transformer is used
- **c** Avoidance of earth leakage currents
- **d** The equipment is earthed
- **e** The equipment meets Class 1 safety standards

88 **An arterial line and its associated measurement system have an intrinsic resonant bandwidth. The system needs to be damped to function correctly and the phrase 'optimal damping' is used to describe the ideal level of damping that should be applied.**

Which of the following statements fits the description of 'optimal damping' most closely?

- **a** Damping where overshoots and oscillations are minimised
- **b** Damping where real-time accuracy is greatest
- **c** Damping where the coefficient is between 0 and 1
- **d** Damping where the response time is greatest
- **e** Damping where there is least resonance

89 **A 55 year-old male with severe symptomatic oesophageal reflux is scheduled for emergency laparotomy for acute small bowel obstruction. Your anaesthetic plan includes rapid sequence induction of anaesthesia. However, at laryngoscopy a Cormack and Lehane grade 3 view is obtained and your initial attempts at intubation are unsuccessful. Facemask ventilation with optimal positioning and a Guedel airway in situ is ineffective and the oxygen saturation has declined to 80%. You call for help urgently.**

Which of the following is the most appropriate immediate course of action whilst awaiting help?

- **a** Insert a laryngeal mask airway and attempt ventilation
- **b** Perform 'asleep' fibreoptic intubation
- **c** Perform cricothyrotomy
- **d** Release cricoid pressure and attempt intubation
- **e** Turn the patient to the left lateral position and allow him to wake up

90 Blood pressure can be measured using an arterial line. The resulting pressure-time curve may be used to estimate several haemodynamic variables.

Which of the following is the best indicator of left ventricular contractility?

- **a** The area under the curve
- **b** The peak of the curve
- **c** The position of the dicrotic notch
- **d** The slope of the upstroke
- **e** The width of the curve

OSCE questions

This section contains twelve examples of the type of OSCE questions used in the Primary FRCA. Some, but not all, are from the RCoA question bank. Each question contains the candidate information, a brief description of the station set-up and for most of the questions, the examiner question sheet.

Dr Campbell Edmondson

Anatomy

Spine

Candidate information:

At this station you will be asked about anatomical features of the spinal cord and its associated functions.

Station set-up:

This station is designed to test the candidate's knowledge of the anatomy and function of the spinal cord.

Questions should be asked as written, using the diagram for the appropriate questions.

For questions 1–3, accept any answer in range given.

1 For a lumbar epidural block, what volume of local anaesthetic is required per segment to be blocked?

2 What is the total CSF volume in the adult?

3 What is the specific gravity of CSF?

4 In a transverse section of the spinal cord, of what is the grey matter composed?

5 On the diagram provided

- (i) Which spinal tracts are represented by the area E (coloured blue)?
- (ii) Which spinal tract is represented by the area F (coloured red)?
- (iii) Which spinal tract is represented by the area C (coloured green)?

6 What type of nerve impulses travel in the corticospinal tracts and how do the fibres terminate?

7 (i) Within the spinal cord, where are ascending pain and temperature fibres carried?

- (ii) Identify the lateral spinothalamic tract on the diagram?

8 What vessels contribute to the arterial blood supply of the spinal cord?

9 What is the origin of the anterior spinal artery?

10 What is the clinical effect of thrombosis of the anterior spinal artery?

COMMUNICATION

Patient anxiety

Candidate guidance:

This station is testing the candidate's communication skills.

You have five minutes with Mrs Anna Foreman, a 55-year-old lady, who is very anxious about her anaesthetic. She is scheduled for a hysteroscopy and has just arrived in theatre.

When you saw her pre-operatively on the ward, you noted that she was well, apart from well-controlled hypertension and occasional angina. She did not mention anxiety. You planned to pre-oxygenate her during induction. The nursing staff in theatre reception have asked you to see Mrs Foreman because she is so anxious and panicky.

Station set-up:

An actress is provided with the following medical history:

You are Mrs Anna Foreman, you are 55, and you have been advised to have a hysteroscopy (a minor procedure) for postmenopausal bleeding. You are worried you may have cancer but are far more worried about the anaesthetic. You had gas for removal of a tooth when you were a child and have been frightened of anaesthetics since. You are frightened of having a mask over your face and of not being able to breathe. You also feel that having an anaesthetic is giving up control and this terrifies you. You think you may have a panic attack.

You saw the candidate earlier when s/he asked you questions about your health. You told them about your high blood pressure and occasional chest pain, both of which are fine as far as you are concerned. You felt rather embarrassed so you did not tell him/her about your anxieties. You did not sleep last night because of your worries and now you are convinced you are going to panic if you have a mask over your face.

You have specific questions for the candidate:

- "What will you do to me?"
- "Do I have to have a mask over my face?"
- "Will I be OK?"

Marks are awarded for the points shown on the answer sheet. At the end of the interview, you should have reached a plan which you and the patient find acceptable.

Equipment

Gas supplies

Candidate information:

You will be shown a photograph of a piece of anaesthetic equipment for delivering gases and be asked questions relating to this subject.

Station set-up:

A picture of an oxygen cylinder (size E) and a Bodock seal are provided for the relevant questions. Any answer within the range provided is acceptable.

1. This is a standard size E oxygen cylinder. What is it made of?
2. Can this cylinder be used in an MRI scanner?
3. If NO, why not?
4. What is the pressure inside a full cylinder of oxygen?
5. What does the Tare weight marked on the cylinder refer to?
6. What is this item of equipment and what does it do?
7. What does it do?
8. What is the pressure in a nitrous oxide pipeline?
9. On an anaesthetic machine, what should be the minimum flow in an oxygen bypass circuit?
10. What is the function of the pressure relief valve on the back bar of an anaesthetic machine?
11. At what pressure does the pressure relief valve on the back bar open?
12. What are the internal and external diameters of the common gas outlet of an anaesthetic machine?
13. What safety mechanisms prevent an incorrect gas coming out of the common gas outlet of an anaesthetic machine?

Hazards

Microshock

Candidate information:
You will be shown a diagram depicting the electrical connections of a patient to a variety of monitoring devices in the operating theatre.

You will be asked questions relating to the hazard of microelectrocution (microshock), electrical safety and the meaning of a number of symbols which appear on electrical devices which are used in the operating theatre.

Station set-up:
The objective of the examiner's questions is to test the candidate's understanding of the principles underlying microelectrocution (microshock), earthing of electrical devices and the interpretation of British Standard symbols for electrical safety. A number of diagrams will be shown to the candidates.

1 What order of magnitude of current passing along an intravenous catheter in contact with the myocardium, as shown here (E), is required to induce ventricular fibrillation?
2 If all this equipment is functioning normally and the patient is not touching metal on the operating table, why is there no risk of microshock?
3 Are the absolute values of the earth potential relative to the mains at points B, C and D the same?
4 The absolute values of the earth potential relative to the mains of 240 volts may vary. By how much?
5 How could the absolute values of the earth potential at points B, C and D be made equal (equipotential)?
6 If a fault developed in the ECG machine resulting in the patient leads being connected to earth, would microelectrocution (microshock) be more or less likely?
7 The symbol G may also be found on electrical equipment in theatre.
8 The symbol A may also be found on electrical equipment in theatre.
9 From this chart (chart 2) identify the meaning of ANY two other symbols.

History

Varicose veins/asthma

Candidate information:

In the following station you will be asked to take a 5 minute history, as at a pre-anaesthetic visit, from Mr Steven Galey, a 54-year-old man who is to undergo bilateral stripping of varicose veins tomorrow.

You should ask any questions you feel will help with his anaesthetic management peri-operatively.

You are NOT required to perform any type of physical examination of the patient.

Station set-up:

An actor is provided with the following information:

You are Steven Galey, a 54-year-old man who has been admitted for bilateral varicose vein stripping on both legs tomorrow. The veins are on the front and sides of your legs (not at the back). You have a history of bronchial asthma which began in your late teens. Your current medication is a Beclomethasone inhaler and you take two puffs twice a day and Salbutamol inhaler two puffs twice a day.

You are prone to chest infections in the winter and whenever you get flu or a cold your asthma becomes worse. You have antibiotics at home (amoxcillin) to take whenever you have any change in colour of the sputum you cough up. You also have a flu vaccination at the beginning of each winter, given to you at the GP's surgery. You are reasonably well at present.

You are allergic to feathers, fur, cats and house dust. This has been proven with skin tests done at the allergy clinic at the hospital. As far as you know you are not allergic to any drugs but you have been told you should not take Propranolol. In 1968 you had an irregular heart beat following a bout of flu in the winter and you were given some Propranolol by your doctor. You remember taking the first dose at the surgery, and noticing that your tongue had gone numb on the way home. You became exceedingly breathless and you do not remember anything until you woke up in the intensive care unit at the local hospital having had a very severe bout of asthma.

This is the only time you have been in hospital with your asthma. You had eczema as a child and it has reappeared at times of stress during your adult life. It seems to have reappeared recently around your right ankle and it is troublesome. The doctor told you that this eczema was related to the varicose veins as it was different from the eczema you have had before. Both your children have hay fever.

You had a general anaesthetic in the dental chair as a child to have some milk teeth removed, but otherwise you have never had an operation. You are not taking any medicines, but you have noticed that if you take aspirin you become more wheezy. You have never smoked. Your teeth are all your own, with no crowns.

Medication:

- Salbutamol 2 puffs twice daily
- Beclomethasone 2 puffs twice a day
- Amoxcillin 500 mg (when required)

Marks are awarded for the points shown on the answer sheet.

Measurement

pH

Candidate information:

You will be asked questions designed to test your understanding of the measurement of blood gas parameters.

Station set-up:

Diagrams are provided with various items marked relating to the questions as appropriate.

1 Which diagram best represents the hydrogen ion or pH electrode?

2 Assuming diagram B is of a pH electrode, what are the items 'A' made of?

3 Why is it necessary to have two electrodes?

4 'B' is the reference electrode, what is the solution?

5 What is the solution in 'C'?

6 What is the item marked 'D'?

7 What connects the two electrodes?

8 The display 'E' reads pH or H^+ concentration, what does it actually measure?

9 The pH electrode is an integral part of the apparatus for measuring which other physiological parameter?

10 The principle of this electrode can be applied to what other measurements?

11 What chemical equation describes the development of an acidosis by CO_2 accumulation?

Monitoring

Pulse oximeter

Candidate information:

You will be asked questions relating to the principles underlying oximetry and the clinical use of a pulse oximeter.

Station set-up:

This station is designed to test the candidate's understanding of the use, limitations and principles of oximetry. Questions should be asked as written, using the pictures and diagrams as necessary.

1 Suggest two pieces of information this device provides?

2 In a normal individual, what is the approximate arterial p02 at point A in graph 1?

3 What name is used to describe point B on graph 1?

4 What use is made of the value of the p50?

5 What other oxygen-carrying compound has a dissociation curve as shown in graph 2?

6 What are the wavelengths of the light emitted from the diodes commonly used in pulse oximeters?

7 How often do the diodes flash?

8 In graph 3, what term is used to describe point A?

9 If you measured the absorption at point A, what parameter would this reflect?

10 How does a pulse oximeter differentiate between arterial, venous and tissue oxygen saturation?

11 Suggest two clinical situations in which a pulse oximeter may be inaccurate?

12 Suggest a common cause for a pulse oximeter tracing such as in Trace 5?

13 What is the main difference between a clinically used pulse oximeter and a laboratory oximeter which allows the laboratory to report levels of carboxyhaemoglobin and other haemoglobins?

Physical examination

Cranial nerves

Candidate information:
In the following station, you will be required to demonstrate how you would perform a physical examination of the third to the twelfth cranial nerves.

You will not be expected to examine the visual fields, perform ophthalmoscopy or visual acuity. Nor are you expected to test smell.

Sensory testing should be limited to light touch only.

You should give a running commentary on what you are doing as you perform the examination.

Station set-up:
An actor and relevant equipment for cranial nerve testing are provided.

If the candidate starts to test the pharyngeal reflex, ask him/her not to perform the test but just to describe how it would be done.

X-RAY

Cervical spine injury

Candidate information:

You are called to casualty, in your District General Hospital. A 20-year-old man has fallen off his motorcycle and presents with pain in his left shoulder and paraesthesia in both hands. He is fully awake and responsive to commands.

A cervical spine X-ray has been taken by the casualty staff prior to your arrival.

Mark the following statements true or false:

All essential disc spaces are visible

The anterior longitudinal ligament is undamaged

The shadow at the tip of 'A' is an abnormality

There is a fracture of the 2nd cervical vertebra

This neck will be stable in flexion

This patient may become apnoeic

He may develop severe retro-pharyngeal swelling

Urgent intubation is essential

Rapid transfer by 'Blue Light' ambulance to a neurosurgical unit is essential

High dose steroids should be given in casualty

Resuscitation

Pulseless electrical activity

Candidate information:

You receive an urgent call to see a patient on the ward who two hours ago had a laparoscopic cholecystectomy. When you arrive, the patient has collapsed and the nurses have started cardiopulmonary resuscitation (CPR, ventilation with a self-inflating bag and mask and chest compressions). An intravenous cannula is in-situ and an ECG rhythm strip has been recorded.

You are expected to treat the patient in accordance with the 2010 ERC/RCUK guidelines.

Station set-up:

The station is set up to display sinus rhythm on the ECG monitor.

1 What would you first need to confirm?

2 The ECG trace from the patient is shown. In the absence of a pulse, what is the diagnosis?

3 Assuming that the rhythm displayed continues to be slow PEA, how would you proceed?

4 What drugs should subsequently be given? How often should the doses be repeated?

5 What reversible factors may be contributing to the failure of this patient to respond?

6 In this patient (who is two hours post-op) which of these reversible factors is most likely to be causing this clinical picture?

7 If the patient responds to fluid resuscitation with the return of a weak pulse, what further actions should you take?

Sim Man

Endobronchial intubation

Candidate information:

A 35-year-man has just been admitted to your intensive care unit following an elective hernia repair during which he aspirated gastric contents.

He is intubated, sedated and ventilated.

You have been called by the unit because his oxygenation is falling despite increasing the inspired concentration of oxygen to 100%.

The monitor shows an ECG trace, direct arterial pressure trace, pulse oximeter trace, end-tidal CO_2 trace and heart rate.

There are also some blood gas results available.

A new CT2 trainee will hand over to you on ITU – it is their first week on ITU. Explain what you are doing and why.

Station set-up:

The examiner is playing the part of a junior CT2 trainee who has called a more senior trainee for help. He/she will rapidly orientate the candidate to the scenario by saying something like 'Assume the patient is sedated with IV agents.'

The opening statement should be something along the lines of 'Here is our patient in ITU. That's his monitor showing his vital signs over there. I'm not happy with his general condition, his saturation is falling despite being on the ventilator.'

Candidate should examine the patient and detect the clinical problem which should be quickly diagnosed. The patient's condition will improve once the tube is pulled back to the correct position.

The examiner will also ask some questions relevant to the scenario.

Technical Skills

Tracheostomy/Tube change

Candidate information:

In the following station, you will be asked about a tracheostomy tube change in a sedated, ventilated ITU patient who had the tracheostomy done two weeks ago. The patient is being enterally fed through a naso-gastric tube.

You will be also asked to demonstrate the procedure on a manikin and asked some general questions about tracheostomy.

Station set-up:

The manikin is set up with a tracheostomy tube in situ with a new replacement tube available, together with a syringe to inflate/deflate the cuff. Make it clear that the candidate is expected to perform the procedure and reiterate the age of the stoma. No bougie or guide wire is needed according to the Intensive Care Society guidelines for the procedure.

1. There are a number of important preparations that you should make before attempting the tube change. Describe four of them (accept any four of these)
2. Having completed your preparations demonstrate how you would carry out the tube change with the equipment provided (i.e. without bougie/guide wire)
3. What pressure should you inflate the cuff to?
4. At what level should a tracheostomy be sited?
5. A tracheostomy bypasses the upper airway. What functions does the upper airway perform?
6. By what volume does a tracheostomy reduce anatomical deadspace in an adult?
7. In addition to regular suctioning how can we prevent blockage of a tracheostomy tube?
8. What type of tracheostomy tube is this?
9. When might you use a variable flange tracheostomy tube?

SOE 1 questions

SOE 1 deals with pharmacology and physiology. The questions are modified from real exam questions and are designed to help guide you towards constructing an acceptable response rather than merely giving a factual answer.

Every candidate presenting at a particular time will get asked the same initial question. The questions will develop from there with supplementary questions, depending upon the response of an individual candidate, but there is guidance for the examiners to ensure each one follows roughly the same course.

For trainers using this section for sample questions, try to use the supplementary items as a guide to further discussion rather than merely individual items to be answered. Try to develop the question as a discussion asking the candidate why and how things occur, and relate principles to clinical practice as much as possible. Steer your questioning to explore the information the candidate has given you to ascertain what has made them present a particular response and what thinking is going on behind them. Candidates often let themselves down as they have not practised explaining things and talking clearly, logically and sensibly.

These questions cover a large area of the curriculum but cannot cover everything. Practice for the exam will need to cover many other areas but the intention here is to give a few examples to highlight exam technique and to help you prepare rather than provide a comprehensive text book. When undertaking SOE practice ensure you give each question five minutes and try three questions for each topic, and ensure each SOE lasts 30 minutes to maximise your exposure to exam conditions.

Dr Tina McLeod/Dr Mark Forrest

Pharmacology

Dr Mark Forrest

Paper 1

Draw a table to compare the physical properties of isoflurane and sevoflurane.

- How do these properties affect their clinical use?
- What is the relevance of the metabolism of these drugs?
- How do the physical properties of Desflurane differ?

What are the effects of age on renal drug elimination?

- What happens to the renal excretion of drugs in old age?
- What are the clinical implications of these changes?
- Can you give some examples? How can we prevent drug toxicity under these circumstances?

How are anti-arrhythmic drugs classified?

- Can the classification be linked to the cardiac action potential?
- What class of anti-arrhythmic is amiodarone?
- What are the side effects of long-term amiodarone use?

Paper 2

What class of drug is vecuronium?

- How does it work at the neuromuscular junction?
- How does its onset of action compare to rocuronium? Why?
- What are its non neuromuscular effects?

How may drug interactions be classified?

- Give an example of a chemical drug interaction relevant to anaesthesia.
- In what ways can drugs interact with pharmacokinetics? Give examples.
- What do the terms synergistic and additive mean?

What drugs are recommended by NICE for the initial treatment of Type II diabetes mellitus?

- How do these drugs reduce plasma glucose?
- What side effects do they have relevant to anaesthesia?
- What other drugs can be used to treat diabetes mellitus?

Paper 3

How are opioid receptors classified?

- What type of receptor are they. How do they modulate their effects?
- Where are they found in the body?
- What are the significant side effects of opioids?

Draw a graph of plasma concentration against time following intravenous injection of a drug. (Assume the drug is only distributed in one compartment.)

- Explain the concepts of half-life, clearance and volume of distribution.
- How can these be derived?
- How would your graph be altered if the drug was distributed in two compartments?

Where in the nephron do diuretic drugs act?

- Which drugs act on the Loop of Henle and how do they work?
- What are the side effects of loop diuretics?
- How do loop diuretics cause hypokalemia?

Paper 4

What is ketamine?

- How does it exert its anaesthetic effect?
- What side effects does it exhibit?
- How do the properties of its isomers differ?

Where does drug metabolism take place?

- What is the chemical aim of drug metabolism?
- How are drugs metabolised by the liver?
- What is the cytochrome P450 system?

How do phenothiazines act as anti-emetics?

- What other receptors do phenothizines act on? What are their effects?
- What other classes of anti-emetics are there?
- How does cyclizine exert its anti-emetic effect?

Paper 5

What factors contribute to the onset of inhalational anaesthesia?

- Explore patient factors.
- What does a blood gas solubility coefficient of 2 mean?
- What are the second gas and concentration effects?

What is an isomer?

- What types of isomerism are there?
- Give examples relevant to anaesthesia.
- What is the clinical relevance of isomerism?

What conditions are treated with carbamazepine?

- How does it exert its anti-epileptic effect?
- How do other anti-epileptics work?
- What are the side effects of carbamazepine?

Paper 6

What drugs can be used to reverse neuromuscular blockade?

- How do the anti-cholinesterases work? Discuss mechanism of enyme inhibition.
- What are the side effects of neostigmine? How are they reduced?
- What is suggammadex?

How can receptors be classified?

- Discuss the classes of receptor.
- What are the different response times. Clinical significance?
- How does the G-protein receptor work?

What is co-amoxiclav?

- How does its spectrum of activity compare to amoxicillin? Why?
- What are the mechanisms of antibiotic resistance?
- How can the spread of antibiotic resistance be minimised?

Paper 7

What is the site of action of benzodiazepines?

- What class of receptor is this? How do benzodiazepines exert their effect?
- What are the indications for benzodiazepines in anaesthesia and critical care?
- What are the potential side effects? What is flumazenil?

Draw a dose response curve for a full agonist.

- What is a log dose response curve and why do we use them?
- Draw log dose response curves for two drugs with different potency at the same receptor.
- Draw a log dose response curve for an antagonist at the same receptor. What would the curve look like if a full agonist was added?

Where are Histamine Type 1 receptors found in the human body?

- What are the actions of antihistamines? Examples?
- How do they work as anti-emetics?
- What are the adverse effects of antihistamines. How can they be reduced?

Paper 8

Describe the mechanism of action of local anaesthetics?

- What factors affect the onset of local anaesthesia?
- What factors affect duration of action? How else may this be altered?
- What structural classes exist? How does structure relate to activity?

What are the causes of inter-patient variability to drugs?

- Discuss physiological variability
- What genetic polymorphisms can affect drug responses?
- What pathological states can affect drug handling?

Which drugs can be used to reduce stomach acidity?

- Mechanisms of action.
- What are their indications in anaesthesia and critical care?
- How would you reduce the risk of reflux prior to anaesthetising an obstetric patient?

Paper 9

Compare the non-anaesthetic effects of isoflurane and desflurane.

- Discuss the effects on the heart and circulation.
- What are the respiratory effects?
- What other effects do they have?

What types of data can be seen in medical research?

- How can this data be displayed graphically?
- What are parametric and non-parametric data?
- What test would you use to compare alcohol consumption between two groups? Why?

How can drugs affect platelet function?

- What drugs can inhibit platelet activation?
- How do aspirin and clopidogrel exert their anti-platelet effect?
- What are the implications of clopidogrel peri-operatively?

Paper 10

What is aspirin?

- How does it produce analgesia?
- How and where is it absorbed?
- How is it metabolised?

Which esterases are relevant to anaesthetic practice?

- How is suxamethonium metabolised?
- How can this process be affected by disease?
- How is esmolol metabolised? What are the clinical implications?

How are red cells prepared and stored for transfusion?

- What storage solutions can be used? Constituents and purpose?
- What temperature should blood be stored at?
- What are the potential adverse effects of blood transfusion?

Physiology

Dr Tina McLeod

Paper 1

Biochemistry: Blood gas analysis

Identify the abnormalities in these arterial blood gases: pH 7.03, $PaCO_2$ 7.3 kPa, PaO_2 7.1 kPa

Pituitary

Describe the anatomical organisation of the pituitary gland

Neurophysiology

What determines the membrane potential of a nerve fibre?

Paper 2

Cerebral blood flow

Draw a diagram to show the relationship between cerebral blood flow and blood pressure

Immune mechanisms

What types of immunity are there?

Respiratory responses

What is the respiratory response to rebreathing 5% CO_2 in oxygen?

Paper 3

Respiratory physiology – hypoxia

Define hypoxia. What are the potential casuses of hypoxia?

Renal

In the kidney, how is glomerular filtrate produced?

Cardiovascular responses

How does the body respond to changes in systemic blood pressure?

Paper 4

Oxygen transport

How is oxygen transported from the lungs to the cells of the tissues?

Vomiting

What function does vomiting serve?

Myocardial performance

Explain the events in the cardiac cycle (You may be given the left ventricular pressure trace to aid your explanation.)

Paper 5

Ventilation and perfusion in the lung

Define ventilation perfusion ratio

Autonomic nervous system

Contrast the sympathetic and parasympathetic nervous systems

Fluids and capillaries

Describe the factors controlling the movement of fluid across the pulmonary capillary walls

Paper 6

Carbon dioxide transport

How is CO_2 transported from the cells to the lungs?

Renal tubule physiology

Using a straight line to represent the length of the convoluted tubule from Bowman's capsule to the start of the Loop of Henle, show the concentrations of glucose, sodium and inulin.

Neuromuscular function

How does release of acetylcholine from an alpha motor neurone lead to muscle contraction?

Paper 7

Action potential

Draw an action potential for a sinoatrial node cell

Neonatal physiology

How does neonatal physiology differ from adult physiology?

Pain

What would happen if you trod on a pin in your bare feet?

Paper 8

Cardiovascular

What is the relationship between BP, SVR and CO?

Metabolism

What are the body's basic metabolic requirements for exercise?

Alveolar gas equation

How can the partial pressure of oxygen in alveolar gas be calculated?

Paper 9

Cardiovascular responses

Describe the physiological responses to the rapid IV infusion of 1 L of normal saline

Glucose metabolism

How does the body handle a glucose load?

Ventilation

During mechanical ventilation what is the effect on $PaCO_2$ of altering minute ventilation?

Paper 10

Cardiac cycle

On a diagram showing a normal ECG trace for two cardiac cycles, draw left ventricular pressure changes first and then aortic pressure changes on the same time axis

Metabolism

Describe the metabolic responses to starvation

Muscle physiology

Describe the structure of a skeletal muscle fibre. Myofibrils, sarcomere as basic unit. Striations: A, I & H bands; Z- and M-lines

SOE 2 questions

SOE 2 deals with clinical and physics/clinical measurement. The questions are modified from real exam questions and are designed to help guide you towards constructing an acceptable response rather than merely giving a factual answer.

Every candidate presenting at a particular time will get asked the same initial question. The questions will develop from there with supplementary questions, depending upon the response of an individual candidate, but there is guidance for the examiners to ensure each one follows roughly the same course.

For trainers using this section for sample questions try to use the supplementary items as a guide to further discussion rather than merely individual items to be answered. Try to develop the question as a discussion asking the candidate why and how things occur, and relate principles to clinical practice as much as possible. Steer your questioning to explore the information the candidate has given you to ascertain what has made them present a particular response and what thinking is going on behind them. Candidates often let themselves down as they have not practised explaining things and talking clearly, logically and sensibly.

These questions cover a large area of the curriculum but cannot cover everything. Practice for the exam will need to cover many other areas but the intention here is to give a few examples to highlight exam technique and to help you prepare rather than provide a comprehensive text book. When undertaking SOE practice ensure you give each question five minutes and try three questions for each topic, and ensure each SOE lasts 30 minutes to maximise your exposure to exam conditions.

Dr Cleave Gass

Dr Chris Leng

Clinical Anaesthesia

Dr Cleave Gass

Paper 1

Airway assessment/difficult intubation

A healthy 35-year-old woman is on your list for an elective laparoscopic cholecystectomy and you find that she can only open her mouth by two fingers' breadth. What further information would you like to know?

Laryngospasm

At the end of the procedure the patient is extubated. Immediately thereafter, she develops severe laryngospasm. How will you assess and manage this situation?

Post-operative nausea and vomiting

Are patients liable to post-operative nausea and vomiting after cholecystectomy?

(Occurrence and prevention of post-operative nausea and vomiting.)

Paper 2

Ten-year-old child presenting for tonsillectomy

A ten-year-old boy presents for elective tonsillectomy. The indication for surgery is excessive snoring and disturbed sleep. He has a history of asthma and takes regular beclometasone diproprionate (Becotide) but is otherwise healthy. He had a cold one week ago, but his parents say he is now fully recovered.

How would you assess this child pre-operatively?

Anaesthetic plan

What is your anaesthetic plan for this child?

Post-operative distress in a child

After handing over the care of the boy to the recovery staff, you are called back because he is extremely distressed. What might be the cause?

(Post-operative care: analgesia and other issues.)

Paper 3

Elective right inguinal hernia repair in a 46-year-old with diabetes

A 46-year-old male, (who has had Type 1 diabetes since the age of 14), has been admitted for repair of a right-sided inguinal hernia. When you meet him he has a normal BP, HR and temperature. He takes atenolol to control his blood pressure.

What important things would you assess at the pre-operative visit?

Sudden convulsion

This patient is transferred to the Post Anaesthetic Care Area and shortly afterwards suffers a convulsion. What is your differential diagnosis? How would you manage this situation?

Management of concurrent medication

What regular medication taken by a patient would you ensure was taken on the day of surgery?

Paper 4

Unrousable 29-year-old emergency admission

You are called to the A&E Department at midnight to attend an 'unrousable' 29-year-old man who has been brought in by his friends from a party where he had collapsed. His breathing is irregular and laboured.

How will you proceed?

He develops neurological signs and needs an urgent CT head scan.

How will you proceed?

Needle stick injury

During your management of this case you suffer a needle stick injury with a needle contaminated with this patient's blood. What action would you take?

Paper 5

Assessment of trauma and multiple injuries

You are called to the A&E department to assist with the care of a 17-year-old who has crashed his motorcycle. He has multiple injuries.

What are the priorities in your resuscitation of this patient?

Examination reveals a rigid abdomen

How would you anaesthetise this patient?

Wrong blood

The surgery is proceeding when it is realised that the patient has been given the wrong blood. What problems may the patient develop as a result?

Paper 6

Hypertensive for hernia repair

You are asked to anaesthetise an obese 54-year-old patient for elective hernia repair. He has hypertension controlled by diuretic medication, but on admission to the ward a nurse records his BP as 165/105 mm Hg. Would you postpone elective surgery with such an admission BP?

ST segment changes on ECG

The patient insists on a GA. Halfway through the procedure you notice marked ST segment changes on the ECG. How do you proceed?

Pre-operative visiting and premedication

Why do we visit patients pre-operatively on the ward?

Paper 7

Emergency laparotomy in an 82-year-old man

An 82-year-old man (previously fit and on no medications) presents for emergency laparotomy for presumed perforated bowel. He has passed a total of 100 ml urine over the last 8 hours. He is alert but slightly breathless when speaking. BP=100/60, pulse 105/min.

Is there anything in his history, which you feel, needs more investigation and management prior to surgery?

Anaesthetic technique and intra-operative event

Following appropriate resuscitation of this patient, how would you proceed with general anaesthesia?

Following induction of anaesthesia, there is a profound drop in BP and a fall in EtCO_2 associated with high ventilating pressures. What do you do?

Why might this patient require ventilation on an ITU?

Paper 8

COPD for hernia repair

A male 76-year-old heavy smoker with severe chronic obstructive pulmonary disease has a right inguinal hernia, which is to be repaired electively. He requests a spinal anaesthetic because a friend of his had one recently for a prostatectomy and he thought it would be 'good for his chest'.

Do you think this will be a suitable choice of anaesthetic?

Anaesthetic technique

How would you establish appropriate spinal anaesthesia for this patient?

Ten minutes after the onset of spinal anaesthesia he becomes very pale and drowsy. What do you do?

Post-operative confusion

Twenty four hours later, you are asked to review the patient on the ward. The ward staff say he has been extremely confused and agitated since the operation. Why might this be?

Paper 9

Obese patient for a hysteroscopy

A 57-year-old lady is listed as a gynaecology day case for a hysteroscopy. You see her on the morning of surgery and discover that she is of average height and weighs 112 kg. She describes recent episodes of chest pain.

What aspects of her history concern you?

Anaesthetic technique

This patient insists on a general anaesthetic. How would you proceed?

Difficulty breathing in recovery

After handing over the care of the patient to the recovery staff, you are called back because she is having difficulty breathing. What might be the cause?

Paper 10

Elective Caesarean section

A 19-year-old primigravida at 39 weeks' gestation is booked for elective Caesarean section because of a transverse presentation.

What are the main anaesthetic issues with such cases?

Difficulty breathing after onset of spinal anaesthesia

You decide to perform a spinal anaesthetic, but after the spinal injection, the patient complains of severe breathing difficulty. What do you do?

Headache

Why might a woman complain of a headache 24 hours after a Caesarean section under spinal anaesthesia?

Physics, clinical measurement, equipment and safety

Dr Chris Leng

Paper 1

Graphical relationships
Show diagrams and ask candidate if they recognise any of them. Go on from there.

Needles used in anaesthetic practice
Show photograph of Tuohy needle – what is this needle used for?

Ask candidate to describe detail of design and relate to function.

pH electrodes
What units do we use to measure the acidity of a blood sample?

Paper 2

Electrical circuit components; defibrillation
Show candidate the card with various electrical symbols. Do you recognise any of those symbols on the card? What are they?

Resuscitation bags and valves
What type of resuscitation bag do you find on a cardiac arrest trolley? How does it work?

Indirect blood pressure measurement
How do you measure blood pressure on the ward?

Paper 3

Freezing point, melting point, latent heat, vapourisation
Could you define the freezing and boiling points of a substance?

Measuring FiO_2 and PO_2
How may the concentration of oxygen in a gas mixture be measured?

Pulse oximetry
How does a pulse oximeter work?

What are the sources of inaccuracy – the effect of different haemoglobins?

Paper 4

Physics of gas laws

A partly used size D oxygen cylinder of volume 2.3 L has a pressure of 100 atmospheres. During transport, for how long could it be used to supply oxygen at 4.6 L min^{-1} into a breathing system?

Principles of measurement

What do you understand by the term calibration? What does an ideal calibration curve look like?

Breathing systems – Mapleson A, C, D, E and F

Show diagram of different breathing systems. How is efficiency gauged in these breathing systems?

Compare the mechanisms behind the efficiency of some of these systems.

Paper 5

Capnography

What does a capnometer measure? What are the principles involved in the measurement?

Bernoulli's principle and Venturi effect

Show the photograph of a ventimask. Can you describe how this works?

Force, energy and work

What do you understand by 'force' and what are its units?

Paper 6

Doppler

Define the Doppler effect, using an equation to help your explanation.

What is duplex Doppler?

What are the medical uses of Doppler?

Cardiac output waveform analysis

What information can be derived from a direct arterial pressure wave?

How can an arterial waveform be used to monitor cardiac output?

Infusion devices

What types of infusion devices are available?

Paper 7

Heat loss during anaesthesia and surgery

How is heat lost during anaesthesia and surgery?

Scavenging systems

What methods are available for reducing the concentration of volatile agents in the theatre atmosphere?

Factors affecting the dynamic response of an arterial line

In what ways may a direct arterial pressure transducer give you false information?

Paper 8

Heat transfer (using blood as an example)

What are the physical principles involved when blood is warmed prior to transfusion?

Electrical hazards

Why is the diathermy pad always checked at the end of an operation?

Temperature measurement

How may a patient's temperature be measured? What physical principles are involved in the measurement?

Paper 9

Principles of magnetism

What equipment employs magnets?

Measurement of biological potentials

What piece of equipment converts biological signals measured in microvolts or millivolts into well reproduced signals in the order of volts?

Types of needle used in anaesthetic practice

What types of needle do you use in your anaesthetic practice?

Paper 10

Electrical components, Ohm's Law, watts, current density

Can you identify the circuit components shown in the diagram?

Measurement of cylinder pressure, pressures up to 1 atmosphere, vacuum

If you had to measure the pressure in a gas cylinder, what instrument would you use?

Disconnection monitors

Which monitors are essential for the induction and maintenance of general anaesthesia?

ANSWERS

3

MCQ answers

MTF Questions 1–20: Pharmacology

1 **a: False.** Cisatracurium is one of the ten stereoisomers present in atracurium.

b: False. It is three to four times more potent than atracurium.

c: False. It does not undergo direct hydrolysis by plasma esterases, but is predominantly eliminated by Hofmann elimination to laudanosine and a monoquaternary acrylate. This is then hydrolysed by non-specific plasma esterases to a monoquaternary alcohol and acrylic acid.

d: True. See above: none of the metabolites of cisatracurium have neuromuscular blocking properties.

e: False. The elimination of both atracurium or cisatracurium is independent of renal function.

2 **a: False.** Propofol is insoluble in water but highly soluble in fat and requires preparation as a lipid emulsion.

b: False. It has a terminal elimination half-life of five to twelve hours.

c: True.

d: False. As well as acting on the β subunit of the GABA receptor it also enhances the effect of glycine which is the major inhibitory transmitter in the brainstem and spinal cord. It also inhibits neurotransmission at excitatory central nicotinic acetylcholine receptors.

e: True. Antagonism of the D2 receptor is a possible mechanism for its anti-emetic effects.

3 **a: False.** Tetracaine (amethocaine) is an ester local anaesthetic.

b: True. Potency is closely related to lipid solubility *in vitro*.

c: False. Rate of onset of action is closely related to pKa. Increasing the dose will increase the absolute amount of unionised drug present and hence increase the speed of onset.

d: True. Ropivacaine is four times more potent than lidocaine, reflecting its greater lipid solubility.

e: False. Cocaine is 95% plasma protein bound.

4 **a: False.** 'Fade' is a feature of partial non-depolarising blockade. Prejunctional nicotinic receptors normally provide positive feedback to maintain transmitter release during periods of high neuromuscular activity; 'fade' may be caused by non-depolarising neuromuscular blocking drugs acting at prejunctional receptors. No 'fade' is seen during tetanic stimulation in the presence of partial depolarisation blockade.

b: True.

c: False. Post-tetanic facilitation is a feature of non-depolarising blockade.

d: False. Small doses of non-depolarising neuromuscular blockers were previously given in an attempt to decrease muscle pains after succinylcholine but have no effect on phase 1 block itself. Phase 1 block may be potentiated by volatile agents, anticholinesterases, magnesium and lithium.

e: False. Dantrolene prevents release of calcium from the sarcoplasmic reticulum and may cause skeletal muscle weakness.

5 **a: True.** Immune mediated heparin-induced thrombocytopaenia is serious and often associated with thrombotic complications. A non-immune thrombocytopaenia also occurs but is rarely of clinical significance.

b: True. This is caused by inhibition of aldosterone secretion.

c: True.

d: False. Heparin has low lipid solubility and does not cross the placenta.

e: True. This is caused by complexing of heparin with mineral substances from bone.

6 **a: True.** Mannitol is a polyhydric alcohol prepared in water as a 10 or 20% solution. The initial increase in circulating volume associated with its administration will reduce the serum sodium concentration by dilution.

b: False. Mannitol increases serum osmolality.

c: True. The initial increase in circulating volume produces an increased preload and cardiac output.

d: False. An increase in extracellular osmolality will draw water out of cells.

e: True. Mannitol is unable to cross the intact blood brain barrier and by virtue of the increased plasma osmolality it draws extracellular brain water into the plasma.

7 **a: True.** Mannitol is an osmotic diuretic. It is freely filtered at the glomerulus but not reabsorbed in the tubules.

b: False. Acetazolamide inhibits carbonic anhydrase. H+ excretion is inhibited and HCO_3- is not reabsorbed, giving alkaline urine.

c: True. Thiazides act mainly on the early portion of the distal tubule inhibiting Na^+ and Cl^- reabsorption.

d: False. Furosemide potentiates aminoglycoside ototoxicity.

e: True. Bumetanide is a loop diuretic.

8 **a: False.** Rifampicin induces hepatic enzymes and antagonises the effect of warfarin.

b: True. Aspirin impairs platelet function, which will potentiate the effects of warfarin. It also competes for plasma binding sites.

c: False. There are no interactions between warfarin and therapeutic doses of paracetamol.

d: True. Amiodarone inhibits warfarin metabolism.

e: True. Tamoxifen inhibits warfarin metabolism.

9 **a: True.** Ketamine is a non-competitive inhibitor of ion channels associated with NMDA receptors.

b: False. Ketamine is a phencyclidine derivative.

c: True. Ketamine has one chiral centre and is presented as a racemic mixture of its two enantiomers, S (+)-ketamine and R (-)-ketamine.

d: True.

e: False. Ketamine causes sympathetic nervous system activation, increases plasma catecholamine concentrations and it thereby produces an indirect positive inotropic effect on the heart. This counteracts the mild direct negatively inotropic effect of ketamine on the heart.

10 **a: False.** Etomidate is ten to twenty times more potent than thiopental.

b: True. Ketamine is demethylated to the active norketamine by hepatic P450 enzymes and then undergoes further glucuronidation.

c: True.

d: False. The hepatic extraction ratio describes the arteriovenous gradient across the liver. It is influenced by liver blood flow, plasma protein binding and hepatic enzyme activity. Drugs with a high extraction ratio such as propofol are readily extracted from blood passing through the liver. Propofol clearance is high and sensitive to changes in liver blood flow. By contrast, thiopental has a low extraction ratio. Clearance is primarily influenced by changes in protein binding and hepatic enzyme activity.

e: True.

11 **a: False.** Benzodiazepines bind to the α-subunit of $GABA_A$ receptors.

b: False. Unlike diazepam and midazolam, the metabolites of lorazepam are inactive.

c: True.

d: False. Benzodiazepines increase the frequency of opening of the $GABA_A$ chloride channel but do not affect plasma chloride.

e: True. At pH >4 the ring structure of midazolam closes, rendering it unionised, lipid soluble and able to cross lipid membranes.

12 **a: True.** Salmeterol binds to the beta-2 adrenoceptor, giving it a duration of action up to twelve hours.

b: True.

c: True. Aminophylline is a non-selective phosphodiesterase inhibitor.

d: True. Salbutamol stimulates beta receptors which are coupled to Gs proteins and activate adenylyl cyclase.

e: True. Salbutamol stimulates Na^+/K^+ ATPase, transferring K^+ from the extracellular to intracellular compartment.

13 **a: True.**

b: False. Alfentanil has a lower clearance than morphine, but a shorter half-life due to its smaller volume of distribution.

c: True. As above, the shorter half-life of alfentanil in comparison to fentanyl is due to its smaller volume of distribution despite lower clearance.

d: False. Fentanyl is approximately ten times more potent than alfentanil.

e: True. Alfentanil is the most protein bound of the opioids at 90%.

14 **a: False.** The effects of cyclizine last four to six hours.

b: False. Cyclizine may have some effect on gastric acid secretion through its anti-cholinergic activity but this is not clinically useful.

c: False. Cyclizine is metabolised by N-demethylation to the inactive molecule norcyclizine.

d: True. In addition to its antihistamine activity cyclizine also has mild anti-cholinergic activity.

e: False. As with most older antihistamines, sedation is a significant side effect.

15 **a: True.** NSAIDs are weak acids that are extensively (up to 99%) protein bound, with a small volume of distribution (0.1 to 0.2 L/kg). Therefore they may potentiate other highly protein bound drugs by displacing them from their binding sites .

b: False. See above.

c: False. COX-1 inhibition impairs prostaglandin production in the gastric mucosa regardless of route of administration.

d: False. Specific COX-2 inhibitors (and some non-specific NSAIDs) are associated with an increased risk of thrombotic events including MI and stroke.

e: False. Reduced thromboxane production inhibits platelet aggregation and adhesion.

16 **a: False.** The boiling point of sevoflurane is 58°C, isoflurane is 48°C.

b: True.

c: True. Sevoflurane is 3.5% metabolised compared to desflurane 0.02%.

d: False. Sevoflurane causes a dose-dependent respiratory depression.

e: True.

17 **a: True.** Stimulation of CNS α2 receptors causes sedation and a reduction in MAC of up to 50%.

b: False. Neostigmine is a quaternary amine and does not cross the blood brain barrier, and therefore has no central effects.

c: True. Amphetamines are powerful central sympathomimetics, and with acute use act as stimulants and increase MAC. However chronic use leads to a reduced anaesthetic requirement, possibly due to depletion of CNS catecholamines.

d: True. Methyldopa decreases MAC by reducing central and peripheral noradrenaline levels.

e: False.

18 **a: True.** Hepatic metabolism of morphine produces active metabolites, including morphine-6-glucuronide, which are subsequently excreted in the urine.

b: True. Ranitidine is partially metabolised in the liver, however 50% is excreted unchanged in the urine.

c: False. Alfentanil is metabolised in the liver to inactive compounds.

d: False. Propofol is metabolised in the liver to inactive compounds.

e: False. Labetalol is metabolised in the liver to inactive compounds.

19 **a: False**. Diamorphine is a synthetic 3,6-diacetyl ester of morphine.

b: True. Unlike morphine, diamorphine is highly lipid soluble.

c: False. Diamorphine is a pro-drug with no affinity for opioid receptors. It is rapidly metabolised in the liver to active 6-monoacetylmorphine and morphine itself.

d: True. High lipid solubility facilitates absorption from subcutaneous tissues.

e: True. See 19c.

20 **a: True.** Soluble insulin acts within 30-60 minutes.

b: False. Insulin glargine consists of hexameric microcrystals at physiological pH, delaying absorption.

c: True. Insulin lispro is a fast-acting insulin analogue with an onset within fifteen minutes.

d: False. Complexing insulin with zinc reduces solubility and delays absorption.

e: False. The addition of protamine causes the insulin to form a hexameric complex, delaying absorption.

MTF Questions 21–40: Physiology

21 **a: False.** Vasopressin, or antidiuretic hormone (ADH), is synthesised in the hypothalamus and secreted by the posterior pituitary.

b: False.

c: True. The anterior pituitary develops as an upgrowth from the primitive mouth (stomatodeum). The posterior pituitary is an extension of the hypothalamus.

d: True. These are probably degranulated secretory cells (chromophils).

e: True. The portal supply links a primary capillary plexus in the hypothalamus to a secondary plexus in the anterior pituitary (AP). Consequently, releasing and inhibitory factors secreted by the hypothalamus reach the AP in higher concentration than if they were secreted into the systemic circulation and presented to the AP via its arterial circulation.

22 **a: False.** Inulin is freely filtered at the glomerulus and will therefore be present in the same concentration.

b: False. In the healthy kidney, the glomerulus is impermeable to large molecules. Albumin (MW 70 000 Da) is not filtered to any significant extent and the glomerular filtrate is essentially protein free.

c: True. Amino acids are freely filtered and filtrate concentration is equal to that of plasma. They are normally completely reabsorbed in the proximal tubule.

d: True. Glucose is freely filtered and completely reabsorbed in the proximal tubule unless the transport maximum is exceeded, e.g. in diabetes.

e: False. Uric acid is filtered at the glomerulus. It is also reabsorbed and secreted by the proximal tubule.

23 **a: True.** Following increased secretion of catabolic hormones.

b: False. Increased aldosterone secretion promotes sodium and water reabsorption from the distal tubule in exchange for potassium excretion.

c: False. This is largely due to changes in endocrine activity outlined below.

d: True. Secondary to increased activity of the hypothalamo-pituitary-adrenal axis.

e: True. Secondary to sympathetic nervous system activation.

24 **a: False.** Minute ventilation increases early in pregnancy, reaching 50% above non-pregnant values at term.

b: False. This is little changed.

c: True. See 24a.

d: True. Caused largely by diaphragmatic elevation as the uterus enlarges.

e: True. Lung compliance remains unchanged, but chest wall compliance decreases as a result of diaphragmatic elevation.

25 **a: True.** Although some auto-immune diseases are examples of hypersensitivity reactions.

b: True.

c: False. Plasma cells are B cells which have been exposed to antigen and secrete large quantities of antibody.

d: False. Antibody production is a humoral response.

e: False. This is a feature of a type I hypersensitivity reaction.

26 **a: True.** The third cranial nerve supplies the levator palpebrae superioris muscle.

b: False. Interruption of the parasympathetic supply to the eye causes mydriasis, or dilatation of the pupil.

c: True. As a result of loss of sympathetic innervation to the superior tarsal muscle. One of the features of Horner's syndrome.

d: False. The fifth cranial nerve supplies the muscles of mastication and provides the sensory supply to the face.

e: False. The supra-orbital nerve, a branch of the frontal nerve, is purely sensory in function.

27 **a: False.** This is due to a relative lack of protein in CSF.

b: False. Hydrogen ion concentration is slightly higher in CSF than in arterial blood.

c: True. See 27a. CSF protein concentration is only about 0.5% that of plasma.

d: True. In order to maintain electrical neutrality. Anionic protein concentration is less than that of blood.

e: False. Glucose concentration is lower in CSF.

28 **a: False.** Portal blood flow exceeds hepatic arterial blood flow by a 2:1 ratio.

b: False. It is at the periphery and forms a triad along with hepatic arterial and portal venous branches.

c: False. See 28a.

d: False. Venous pressures as high as this are pathological (portal hypertension).

e: True. At the periphery of the lobule, portal venous and hepatic arterial blood mix to flow along sinusoids towards the centre of the lobule. The centre is most vulnerable in low perfusion states or hypoxia (centrilobular necrosis).

29 **a: False.** This is unchanged.

b: True. When glucose is completely metabolised, $C_6H_{12}O_6 + 6O_2 \rightarrow 6CO_2 + 6H_2O$, the respiratory quotient, RQ, the ratio of the volume of carbon dioxide produced to oxygen consumed, is one. RQ decreases during starvation as alternative, more reduced, energy sources are used (see below).

c: True. In order to promote gluconeogenesis.

d: True. Glucose production switches from glycogenolysis to gluconeogenesis from non-carbohydrate sources. Amino acids are mobilised from muscle and are deaminated during gluconeogenesis.

e: False. Free fatty acids are an important energy source and in addition, production of ketone bodies such as acetoacetic acid and ß-hydroxybutyric acid increases, leading to acidosis.

30 **a: True.** Intracellular sodium concentration (15 $mmol.L^{-1}$) is much less than extracellular (140 $mmol.L^{-1}$).

b: False. Active reabsorption of sodium and other solutes decreases the osmotic pressure of tubular fluid and passive water reabsorption occurs down the osmotic gradient.

c: False. In the presence of ADH, the wall of the collecting duct (CD) becomes permeable to water, allowing water to passively follow the osmotic gradient between CD and medullary interstitium, which has very high osmolarity.

d: True. The process known as iodide trapping.

e: True. Via a H^+/K^+ ATPase (proton pump). There is a 10^5-10^6-fold hydrogen ion concentration gradient between parietal cells (pH 7.3 or so), and the gastric lumen (pH 1-2). ($pH = -log_{10}[H^+]$).

31 **a: False.** Dietary protein is broken down into amino acids for absorption in the small intestine.

b: False. In health, protein is not filtered at the glomerulus in significant quantities.

c: False. Albumin is a non-specific carrier for a variety of substances such as bilirubin, fatty acids, thyroid hormone, calcium and drugs.

d: False. Immunoglobulins are the proteins with antibody properties.

e: True.

32 **a: False.** Closing capacity (CC) equals residual volume plus closing volume.

b: False. It is attributable to collapse of smaller airways.

c: True.

d: False. It is measured by measuring nitrogen concentration in expired gas following a vital capacity breath of 100% oxygen. An abrupt increase in nitrogen concentration at the onset of phase 4 occurs as a result of preferential emptying of apical units and represents the volume of the lung at which dependent airways begin to close.

e: False. However, FRC increases on moving from supine to standing and CC is then less liable to encroach on FRC.

33 **a: True.** The partial pressure of oxygen at which haemoglobin is 50% saturated is a measure of the affinity of haemoglobin for oxygen and can be readily plotted on the curve.

b: False. Oxygen carrying capacity is determined primarily by haemoglobin concentration.

c: False. Red cell 2,3-DPG is increased in anaemia, shifting the curve to the right, facilitating the offloading of oxygen at cellular level.

d: False. The carboxyhaemoglobin (COHb) curve is hyperbolic rather than sigmoid shaped. In the presence of COHb, the dissociation curve of the remaining HbO_2 shifts to the left. In addition, haemoglobin has an affinity for CO 200 times that of O_2 and COHb releases CO very slowly.

e: True. Hyperventilation causes respiratory alkalosis and shifts the curve to the left.

34 **a: True.**

b: False. Resistance = Pressure difference between alveoli and mouth per unit of airflow (compare electrical resistance: R =V/I), so the units are $kPa.s.L^{-1}$.

c: False. As lung volume is reduced, airway resistance increases markedly. At low lung volumes, small airways may close completely, especially in dependent parts of the lung.

d: True. Airway compression occurs with increasing intra-thoracic pressure.

e: False. Airway resistance increases as flow changes from laminar to turbulent.

35 **a: True.** $PaCO_2$ decreases secondary to hyperventilation.

b: False. See a., above. pH = pKa + $\log_{10}[HCO3^-]/\alpha PaCO_2$.
To compensate for the respiratory alkalosis, hydrogen ion is conserved and bicarbonate is excreted in urine, decreasing plasma bicarbonate concentration to maintain the bicarbonate/CO_2 concentration ratio and restore plasma pH towards normal.

c: True. Hypoxia causes an increase in pulmonary vascular resistance (hypoxic pulmonary vasoconstriction).

d: True. In an attempt to maintain oxygen delivery or flux.

e: False. This is a longer term response.

36 **a: True.** Myocardial oxygen consumption is determined primarily by heart rate, contractility and intra-myocardial tension.

b: True. See above. Ventricular work correlates with oxygen consumption.

c: True. See a and b, above.

d: True. This can substitute for fibre length in Starling's Law of the heart.

e: True. See 36d. An increase in PCWP corresponds to an increase in preload.

37 **a: False.** The coronary sinus drains into the right atrium.

b: True. Some Thebesian veins drain directly into the left side of the heart.

c: False. The anterior cardiac veins drain the anterior part of the right ventricle, opening into the right atrium.

d: True. Although the bronchial veins drain into the azygous systems, the majority of bronchial venous drainage is via the pulmonary veins, thus contributing to shunt.

e: False. The ductus venosus is an embryological structure connecting the umbilical vein to the inferior vena cava, allowing about 50% of oxygenated blood to bypass the liver.

38 **a: False.** Hypoxia increases intracranial pressure and is a cause of secondary brain injury.

b: True. Intracranial pressure increases as $PaCO_2$ increases.

c: True. Coughing and straining increase intracranial pressure.

d: False.

e: False. This technique is used to measure cerebral blood flow.

39 **a: False.** Aldosterone promotes both sodium and water reabsorption.

b: True. ADH increases water reabsorption in collecting ducts.

c: False. Cortisol has weak mineralocorticoid activity.

d: True. Dehydration increases ADH secretion from the posterior pituitary in response to increased hypothalamic osmoreceptor activity.

e: True. Urinary nitrogen excretion is increased, increasing the number of osmotically active particles.

40 **a: True.** This is a lower motor neurone lesion. Intact anterior horn cells are required for the efferent limb of the tendon reflex.

b: False. Corticospinal tract damage is an upper motor neurone (UMN) lesion, leading to weakness, increased muscle tone and increase in tendon reflexes.

c: False. This UMN lesion would cause an increase in tendon jerks and in muscle tone (e.g. following a stroke).

d: False. See 40c.

e: False. These are ascending sensory fibres.

MTF Questions 41–60: Physics, Clinical Measurement and Statistics

41 **a: False.** The tip of the catheter should be within superior vena cava and that distance will vary between patients.

b: False. The usual adult size catheters are 14-16 Gauge, corresponding to 1.63 and 1.3 mm diameter.

c: True. Either internal jugular or subclavian vein could be used as long as the catheter tip is located in the superior vena cava.

d: True. Microshock is a term describing the induction of ventricular fibrillation by small electrical currents (below the threshold of skin sensation, i.e. below 1 mA) when applied to very small areas of ventricular muscle, usually by vascular catheters or wires. It requires a small area of contact with heart muscle so that the current density is high despite low current.

e: False. It is usually set at the point where the fourth intercostal space and mid-axillary line cross each other. This allows the measurement to be as close to the right atrium as possible with the patient in a supine position.

42 At this point an inhalational agent will be at its saturated vapour pressure (SVP). It is only the temperature of the liquid that influences the SVP. The higher the temperature, the higher the SVP. Hence, the only correct answer is D.

a: False.

b: False.

c: False.

d: True.

e: False.

43 **a: False.** Pascal is the SI unit of pressure. 1Pa=1N m^{-2} . Force is expressed in Newtons. 1N=1kg m s^2: A force of 1 N will give a mass of 1 kg an acceleration of 1 m per second.

b: False. The SI unit of mass is the kilogram.

c: True.

d: True.

e: False. Watt is a derived unit of power (the rate of doing work, J S^{-1}). The unit of energy is Joule. 1J =1Nm. One Joule is the energy expended when the point of application of a force of 1N moves 1m in the direction of the force.

44 **a: True.** This is a definition of critical temperature.

b: True.

c : False. At the very end of its use, there is no liquid left in the cylinder only vapour. This is when the pressure in the cylinder starts to drop rapidly. In addition, at temperatures above its critical temperature the cylinder will contain only gas.

d: False. The critical temperature of nitrous oxide is 36.5°C.

e: False. The critical pressure of a substance is the pressure required to liquefy a gas at its critical temperature.

45 **a: True.** Boyle's Law is an ideal gas law and assumes among other things that molecular size is unimportant

b: True. This is the definition of Boyle's Law

c: False. Charles' Law states that at a constant pressure, the volume of a given mass of gas varies directly to its absolute temperature. Absolute temperature is measured in Kelvin. 0°C = 273K. Hence, 10°C= 10+273=283K and 20°C=20+273=293K. So, when temperature rises from 10 to 20°C the pressure only goes up by 3.5% (it does not double). The temperature change in Kelvin is only 10K (10K is 3.5% of the initial 283K).

d: False. Dalton's Law states that in a mixture of gases, the pressure exerted by each gas is equal to the pressure which would be exerted if that gas alone were present. Hence, the total pressure exerted by the mixture of gases is equal to the sum of the partial pressures of individual gases.

e: False. Laplace's Law for spheres reads $P= 2T/R$, where P is the pressure gradient across the wall, T is the tangential force acting along the length of the wall and R is the radius. So in large alveoli, the radius will be larger and consequently the resultant pressure gradient across the wall will be smaller. That is why large alveoli do not collapse and there is a tendency of small alveoli to empty into large alveoli. In normal lungs this does not occur due to the presence of surfactant lining the alveoli.

MCQ

46 **a: True.** The Doppler effect for electromagnetic waves such as light is invaluable in astronomy. It has been used to measure the speed at which stars and galaxies are approaching or receding from us.

b: False. It is the change of frequency of a signal that is key to the Doppler effect.

c: False. That is the true of clinical ultrasound but not the Doppler effect.

d: True. And the opposite is correct showing the shift to a higher frequency if the source is moving towards the receiver.

e: True. The sound waves reflect from surfaces of the red blood cells as they approach and move away. Analysis of the reflected frequencies allows determination of velocity of flow.

47 **a: True.** The refractometer, sometimes called the interferometer can measure the concentration of any inhalational agent. It measures the extent to which light is bent (i.e. refracted) when it moves from air into a sample.

b: False.

c: False. It absorbs infrared radiation.

d: True. That is the principle of infrared analyser when used to measure the concentration of sevoflurane and other substances containing two dissimilar atoms in a molecule.

e: True. Mass spectrometry works by ionising chemical compounds to generate charged molecules or molecular fragments. Their mass-to-charge ratios are then measured.

48 **a: False.** The inner tube carries the fresh gas flow. By contrast, the coaxial Mapleson A system (Lack) carries the fresh gas flow in the outer tube.

b: False. Rebreathing would definitely occur at a fresh gas flow equal to minute ventilation. To prevent rebreathing, a fresh gas flow of 2-4 times per minute ventilation is usually quoted.

c: True. In fact, it has been safely used in children weighing less than 20 kg.

d: True. Apparatus dead space is that volume of a breathing system that contains alveolar gases that are inhaled on a subsequent breath. Following this disconnection, it is increased. Alveolar gases would be pushed towards (rather than away from) the patient by the fresh gas flow risking dangerous accumulation of carbon dioxide.

e: False. It is Mapleson D. The Mapleson classification is specific about the spatial relationship between fresh gas flow input, reservoir bag, APL valve and tubing in the system.

49 **a: True.** Nitrous oxide, oxygen and medical air are all supplied at a pipeline pressure of 4.1 Bar.

b: True. As the pressure within the in-use bank of cylinders falls, a passive shuttle is pushed over by the higher pressure within the adjacent full cylinder bank and a continuous downstream pressure is maintained. No power supply is required, other than to sound an alarm.

c: True. For safety, the collars are pipeline specific and non-interchangeable. Alongside non-interchangeable screw threads (NIST) on pipeline connections and the pin index system on cylinder yokes, they are key to the safe delivery of the correct gases through an anaesthetic machine.

d: True. The outlets feature on both the positive pressure gas and sub atmospheric vacuum pipelines.

e: False. An oxygen analyser would detect the presence of oxygen, but not the maintenance of pressure within the pipeline. The latter would also be needed to comment on the integrity of the system.

50 **a: False.** Unpaired electrons in the outer shell are needed for paramagnetism. Therefore, magnesium, lithium, molybdenum and tantalum also exhibit paramagnetism.

b: False. The glass spheres are full of nitrogen which is weakly diamagnetic (slightly repelled by the magnetic field).

c: True. The tension of suspending ligament determines the orientation of the dumb-bell in the magnetic field.

d: True. In this device, photocells are used to control a variable current that induces a magnetic field that exactly offsets the movement due to the paramagnetic effect of the oxygen. The current is used to calculate the oxygen concentration.

e: True. Water vapour affects the accuracy of many gas analysers including the paramagnetic gas analyser. The water vapour can also coat the internal mechanism.

51 **a: True.** In contrast to laminar flow and transitional flow (at the Reynolds number), viscosity changes do not affect established turbulent flow.

b: True. Plasma protein concentration and haematocrit are the two key determinants of blood viscosity. Pathological increases in plasma proteins (such as seen in multiple myeloma) cause a hyperviscosity syndrome.

c: True. The Hagen-Poiseuille equation states that laminar fluid flow exhibits a reciprocal relationship with viscosity.

d: True. This relationship is true of most liquids.

e: False. It is the density of helium that is most important. (See the above answer to 51a.)

52 **a: True.** 1 kPa = 1000 Nm^{-2}, 0.01 Bar, 0.01 atmospheres, 7.5mm Hg and 10.2 cm H_2O.

b: True. As above.

c: False. It is essential that the top be open to allow pressure measurement relative to a constant atmospheric pressure. A manometer therefore measures gauge pressure.

d: True. Compared to a manometer, a barometer specifically measures atmospheric pressure. Therefore, the top is closed to allow generation of a Torricellian vacuum. This allows absolute ambient pressure to be measured by the height of the mercury column.

e: True. The word 'aneroid' means 'no liquid'.

53 **a: True.** PEFR shows a nocturnal and early morning dip of up to 10%. A diurnal variation of 20% and above has been suggested as a useful indicator of asthmatic tendency.

b: False. A peak flow meter is more appropriate. A Vitalograph could be used in theory, but is bulky and would require subsequent analysis of its graphical output.

c: False. It is a variable orifice device.

d: False. A rapid capnograph only measures partial pressure of carbon dioxide against time and not gas flow or volume. In any event, the physiological dead space volume of expiration would not be detected.

e: True.

54 **a: True.** This is the definition of a transducer.

b: False. Their only function is to convert one form of energy to another. They cannot therefore increase it. To amplify a signal, a separate amplification system is required.

c: True. Active transducers generate electric current or voltage directly in response to environmental stimulation. (For example thermocouples and piezoelectric accelerometers.) Passive transducers produce a change in a passive electrical quantity, such as capacitance, resistance, or inductance, as a result of stimulation. (For example strain gauges, resistance temperature detectors and thermistors.)

d: False. See answer 54b.

e: True.

55 **a: False.** Inulin is used to measure ECF volume (as well as GFR).

b: False. Deuterium oxide or tritium are isotopes of water, so can be used to measure total body water; ECF volume can be subtracted from this to give ICF volume.

c: True. ICF volume cannot be measured directly, so must be inferred from extracellular and total body water.

d: True. Albumin is a large molecule which stays in plasma.

e: True. ^{51}Cr is an isotope that can be used to tag RBCs; thereby it can be used to calculate RBC volume.

56 **a: False.** Steel alloy cylinders are made of either manganese molybdenum steel, chromium molybdenum steel or nickel chromium molybdenum steel.

b: True. Nitrous oxide is stored in cylinders below its critical temperature, so is a vapour in equilibrium with its liquid.

c: False. Filling ratio is the weight of the cylinder contents divided by the weight of water it could hold.

d: False. The ratio in UK is 0.75.

e: True. Adiabatic expansion of the gas being released at high flow rate will result in the gas cooling and therefore the cylinder will cool as well.

57 **a: False.** The power of a trial is the probability of avoiding a type II statistical error (when the null hypothesis is incorrectly accepted). A power of 80% is required in a well designed trial.

b: False. Double blinding means both investigators and participants are unaware of the nature of the treatment.

c: True. Pilot studies are used for this purpose before committing to the expense of a larger trial.

d: False. A wide confidence interval means that there is less confidence that a variable under study lies within a well defined range; a well designed trial will therefore possess narrow confidence intervals.

e: True. The Chi Squared test is designed to test the difference between expected and observed observations and therefore lends itself to testing differences in sex distribution in a well designed trial.

58 **a: False.** Standard deviation (SD) describes the scatter in the observations around their mean value, and says nothing about bias.

b: False.

c: True. This is the definition of SD.

d: True. In a normally distributed population, 68.3 % of the values lie within 1 SD of the mean, 95.4% lie within 2 SD, and 99.7% lie within 3 SD of the mean.

e: True. The SEM is the SD/√(number in sample), so SD > SEM.

59 **a: False.** The range is 0 to 10.

b: False. This is clearly an asymmetric distribution skewed towards lower values.

c: True. As there are an even number of observations, the median (the middlemost value) is the average of the two either side of the hypothetical middle value.

d: True. The distribution is negatively skewed.

e: False. The most frequent observation in this sample is 1 (three observations), all the other values occur once only; the sample is therefore a skewed, unimodal set, not bimodal.

60 **a: False.** Wetting the skin reduces its electrical impedance and increases the risk of shock.

b: False. Although 24 V AC or 50 V DC are the upper values in Class 3 (low voltage) electrical equipment, and macroshock is unlikely, it is not impossible and does not preclude microshock.

c: True. The principle of electrical safety is to prevent leakage currents to earth. The diathermy plate could form an electrical pathway to earth for a leakage current from any circuit with a patient attachment, not just the diathermy circuit. So modern thinking precludes earthing.

d: True. Microshock, which is shock from an electrical contact placed within the body, can cause ventricular fibrillation at currents above 100 microamps.

e: True. There are a number of causes of leakage current. All current carrying conductors have an associated magnetic field; a changing magnetic field from an alternating current induces a voltage in neighbouring conductors, which may be the cause of an unintended leakage current.

SBA Questions 61–90

61 **Correct answer D.**

Although this scenario describes a probable acute coronary syndrome (ACS), insufficient clinical information is given to be certain of this. Oxygenation of the myocardium is the most important immediate goal as the patient is cyanosed. GTN may exacerbate hypotension. Aspirin and clopidogrel should be given as soon as possible if a diagnosis of ACS is confirmed (and they are not contraindicated) to prevent further thrombus formation but are not the immediate priority. Fibrinolysis is reserved for STEMI and new LBBB. ALS guidelines state that nifedipine should be avoided in ACS.

62 **Correct answer A.**

Although there are several causes of hyperglycaemia in critically ill patients including the stress response, insulin resistance and TPN, an adrenaline infusion is the most likely drug from the list given to cause increased blood glucose, by stimulating glycogenolysis, gluconeogenesis and lipolysis.

63 **Correct answer E.**

The key point is rapid offset of alfentanil. Its smaller volume of distribution means that it has a shorter elimination half-life than fentanyl despite its lower clearance. B is also true of fentanyl. C relates to speed of onset which is useful but not the best reason for using the drug.

64 **Correct answer B.**

The most likely reason for bronchospasm after a NSAID in an asthmatic is over-production of leukotrienes, caused by COX inhibition and shunting of arachidonic acid metabolism away from prostaglandin production.

65 **Correct answer A.**

The maximum recommended safe dose of bupivacaine is 2mg kg^{-1}, either plain or with added adrenaline. B and D are therefore immediately excluded. A and C both contain a safe dose of levobupivacaine 25 mg, as does E with a dose of 22.5 mg. The higher concentrations are unnecessary and more likely to lead to motor weakness. A is a better choice as the greater volume of approximately 1 ml kg^{-1} is more likely to ascend high enough from the level of injection to cover the site of surgery effectively (iliohypogastric and ilioinguinal nerves; T11 and T12 intercostal nerves).

66 **Correct answer E.**

Diamorphine hydrolysis is catalysed by abundant plasma esterases. 6-monoacetylmorphine is an active metabolite, which is further metabolized to morphine. Morphine is metabolised in the liver by glucuronidation to morphine-3-glucuronide and morphine-6-glucuronide. Impaired renal excretion and accumulation of morphine-6-glucuronide, which is thirteen times more potent than morphine with a similar half-life, is a potential hazard when morphine (or diamorphine) is given by infusion to patients with renal failure.

67 **Correct answer A.**

The correct answer is based on the Bowman principle: lower potency requires a larger clinical intubating dose, which means more molecules of the drug are given and so onset is faster according to the law of mass action. B is therefore false. Fasciculation is associated with the use of depolarising neuromuscular blockers. Recovery will be dependent on metabolism. Reversal by sugammadex may be a feature but is not the most predictable property.

68 **Correct answer C.**

The ideal pharmacokinetic properties required of such a marker drug are: 100% oral bioavailability, zero absorption from the stomach and rapid absorption from the small intestine. Gentamicin, vancomycin and propranolol have poor oral bioavailability. Aspirin will be absorbed from the stomach even if gastric emptying is delayed. Paracetamol is well and rapidly absorbed from the small intestine and is often used as a marker of gastric emptying.

69 Correct answer C.

Onset time depends on the concentration gradient between unbound, unionised drug in blood and the brain: a higher lipid solubility will favour a faster onset but this drug is less lipid soluble (lower potency than fentanyl). It has similar protein binding, so similar unbound fraction; clearance is similar to that of fentanyl. The main difference is the lower pKa so a higher unionised fraction.

70 Correct answer B.

The ECG suggests complete heart block with broadened QRS indicating increased risk of asystole. Following ALS guidelines initial treatment of this bradycardia is atropine; pacing may be the next treatment. Glucagon may be indicated if beta-blocker or calcium channel blocker overdose is suspected. An adrenaline infusion may be indicated if atropine fails to restore sinus rhythm and there is a delay in establishing temporary transvenous pacing.

71 Correct answer C.

The renal clearance of a drug is the notional volume of plasma completely cleared of drug by renal excretion per unit time. Hence, renal clearance = amount of drug excreted in urine per unit time divided by plasma concentration.

$$= \frac{[U] \times V}{[P]} = \frac{2500\ \mu g.mL^{-1} \times 1\ mL.min^{-1}}{25\ \mu g.mL^{-1}}$$

72 Correct answer A.

All of the factors listed are influenced by loading conditions (preload, afterload) and/or compliance of LV. Ejection fraction is least influenced and is the best overall measure of contractility in this list.

73 Correct answer E.

The ECG changes are suggestive of an infarct of the inferior left ventricle. The right coronary artery supplies the inferior left ventricle in 90% of the population.

74 **Correct answer D.**

Whilst all of these factors operate, relaxation of the precapillary sphincters (autoregulatory change effected by local mediators) causes skeletal muscle blood flow and hence oxygen supply to increase 20-30-fold. The increase in cardiac output is 'only' 5-10-fold. Oxygen offload from haemoglobin may increase 2-3-fold. The partial pressure gradient for oxygen increases less than 2-fold.

75 **Correct answer E.**

The Haldane effect describes the increased capacity of deoxyhaemoglobin to carry CO_2 as carbaminohaemoglobin and to buffer H^+ ions (histidine residues pKa 6.8) generated from the dissociation of carbonic acid. This is termed isohydric buffering. Plasma proteins and dissolution of CO_2 play a minor role in CO_2 transport. Carbonic anhydrase is of course essential and plays a major role but it cannot buffer pH changes caused by addition of CO_2. The Bohr effect is irrelevant.

76 **Correct answer B.**

All listed changes occur. By far the most important is decreased FRC, which may now encroach on the closing volume, tending to cause an increase in shunt and hypoxaemia. It will also decrease the store of oxygen in the lungs.

77 **Correct answer D.**

Oxygen flux = CO x CaO_2. CO increases by approximately 50% at term. The main reasons for this increase are increased circulating volume (oestrogen effect) and venodilatation (progesterone effect) causing increased venous return. The increased venous return necessitates increased cardiac output. This is a situation somewhat analogous to optimising oxygen delivery using oesophaegal Doppler monitoring to guide fluid loading during surgery in high risk patients. The mechanism for increasing oxygen delivery is increased cardiac output, which is itself dependent on increased preload (increased venous return). None of the other statements is true. There is little or no change in myocardial contractility during pregnancy. Although the RBC mass is increased by 20%, haematocrit falls. There is little change in PaO_2. Position of the oxyhaemoglobin curve is irrelevant to a consideration of oxygen delivery.

78 **Correct answer D.**

This question simply tests knowledge of the Goldman & Nernst equations and that the resting membrane is relatively impermeable to sodium.

79 **Correct answer D.**

SVR is approximately ten times PVR and is mainly at arteriolar level. It is calculated from MAP and CVP: SVR = k x (MAP-CVP)/CO.

80 **Correct answer B.**

The central chemoreceptors are more important than the peripheral chemoreceptors in determining the ventilatory response to carbon dioxide. They are directly sensitive to changes in pH.

81 **Correct answer B.**

Oxygen concentration = $\frac{(6 \times 1.0) + (60 \times 0.21)}{66}$ = 0.282 i.e. ≈ 28%.

82 **Correct answer D.**

Although all of the leaves are true statements, the key reason why the vapouriser functions independently of altitude is that the vapouriser delivers a fixed partial pressure, independent of altitude. B is a variation on D but is less able to explain the phenomenon. For example, if the ambient pressure is 0.5 atm, the delivered concentration is 2% at a dial setting of 1%. This follows from the fact that the SVP of volatile is unchanged at altitude and the splitting ratio remains unchanged.

83 **Correct answer B.**

Lower frequency (longer wavelength) ultrasound waves penetrate to a greater depth – at the expense of decreased resolution.

84 **Correct answer D.**

Although all statements except E are true, the reason the bobbin comes to rest is an expression of Newtonian physics where a stationary body must have equal and opposite forces applied to it. The other statements do not explain why it is brought to rest. None of the other statements can in themselves explain why the bobbin does not continue to rise in the gas flow.

85 **Correct answer C.**

All of the statements are true. However, only C gives a full explanation as to why the cylinder contents are independent of the pressure gauge reading.

86 **Correct answer B.**

The soda lime is exhausted. Clearly this needs to be replaced. However, the most sensible immediate course of action is to increase FGF and to eliminate rebreathing of expired CO_2 and normalise end-tidal CO_2 pending soda lime canister replacement. Increasing minute ventilation will not avoid rebreathing of expired CO_2. This is not MH, which would not normally be associated with a raised baseline on the capnograph.

87 **Correct answer C.**

The whole rationale of electrical safety centres around avoidance of earth leakage currents. A and B are true statements but subsets of C D may or may not be true. E is true for domestic appliances, but is not considered adequate for electromedical devices.

88 **Correct answer B.**

Optimal damping is the trade-off between response (rise) time and overshoot of the true value or resonance. C is true of damping in general, but not of optimal damping. D is true of a very small damping value, but it would oscillate around the true value for too long. E is not best answer, as although lack of resonance is a desirable general property of a measurement system, it is not a feature unique to optimal damping. A is not correct as higher values than 0.7 would cause even fewer overshoots and oscillations, but would have an unacceptably long response time before reaching the true value. B is the best answer, combining minimal oscillation and overshoot, and resistance to resonance across a wider bandwidth of input oscillations.

89 **Correct answer A.**

DAS guidelines should be followed. A laryngeal mask may be effective, without the added risks of removing cricoid pressure (as in option D) – the patient described would be at particularly high risk of regurgitation and aspiration. Briefly reducing cricoid pressure during insertion of the LMA may be considered. Fibreoptic intubation will take too long, cricothyrotomy is unnecessarily invasive at this stage, but may be a last resort. E is dangerous in an apnoeic, obstructed, hypoxic patient.

90 **Correct answer D.**

Myocardial contractility is indicated by the rate of pressure change per unit time (dP/dT), i.e. the slope of the upstroke. The area under the curve reflects stroke volume. The peak is the systolic pressure. The position of the dicrotic notch reflects fluid status and aortic compliance/elasticity. The width of the curve reflects duration of ventricular systole.

OSCE answers

The answers are in italics

ANATOMY

Spine

1 For a lumbar epidural block, what volume of local anaesthetic is required per segment to be blocked?
1.5–2.0 ml

2 What is the total CSF volume in the adult?
100 – 200 ml

3 What is the specific gravity of CSF?
1003 – 1009 (accept 1.003 – 1.009)

4 In a transverse section of the spinal cord, of what is the grey matter composed?
Nerve cell bodies and unmyelinated axons

5 On the diagram provided

(i) Which spinal tracts are represented by the area E (coloured blue)?
Spino-cerebellar tracts (anterior and posterior)

(ii) Which spinal tract is represented by the area F (coloured red)?
Anterior corticospinal tract

(iii) Which spinal tract is represented by the area C (coloured green)?
Lateral corticospinal tract

6 What type of nerve impulses travel in the corticospinal tracts and how do the fibres terminate?
Descending motor impulses
They synapse with motor neurones in the anterior horn

7 (i) Within the spinal cord, where are ascending pain and temperature fibres carried?
Lateral spinothalamic tract

(ii) Identify the lateral spinothalamic tract on the diagram
Coloured pink

8 What vessels contribute to the arterial blood supply of the spinal cord?
Anterior spinal artery
Posterior spinal artery
Any one from radicular arteries or spinal branches of vertebral, intercostal, lumbar or sacral arteries

9 What is the origin of the anterior spinal artery?
Branch from each of the vertebral arteries

10 What is the clinical effect of thrombosis of the anterior spinal artery?
Loss of motor and most sensory modalities with sparing of proprioception and touch (dorsal columns)

Communication

Patient anxiety

Marks awarded for the following:

1. Candidate introduces themselves to patient and is polite
2. Listens to and acknowledges patient's anxiety
   Elicits reason for anxiety (past GA with facemask as a child)
3. Explain compromises available
   Premedication
   Pre-oxygenation not essential
   Holding mask herself
   Explains why oxygen is useful at induction
   Keep mask above face
4. Reassures patients about very low incidence of problems
5. Asks what patient wishes and gives them some control
6. Reaches satisfactory outcome
7. Uses clear English and avoids jargon
8. Has empathy with patient, e.g. good eye contact and body language

Equipment

Gas supplies

1 This is a standard size E oxygen cylinder. What is it made of?
Molybdenum steel

2 Can this cylinder be used in an MRI scanner?
No

3 If NO, why not?
Ferromagnetic and would be drawn into the scanner

4 What is the pressure inside a full cylinder of oxygen?
13,700 kPa (accept 135 atm or 137 Bar or 1980 psi)

5 What does the Tare weight marked on the cylinder refer to?
Weight of the empty cylinder

6 What is this item of equipment?
Bodok seal

7 What does it do?
Prevents a leak of gas between a gas cylinder and the cylinder block

8 What is the pressure in a nitrous oxide pipeline?
420 kPA (allow 400 kPA or 4 Bar)

9 On an anaesthetic machine, what should be the minimum flow in an oxygen bypass circuit?
30 litres/min (allow 35 l/min)

10 What is the function of the pressure relief valve on the back bar of an anaesthetic machine?
To prevent damage to the vapourisers
To prevent damage to the rotameters (NOT patient)

11 At what pressure does the pressure relief valve on the back bar open?
30 to 40 kPA

12 What are the internal and external diameters of the common gas outlet of an anaesthetic machine?
15 mm and 22 mm

13 What safety mechanisms prevent the wrong gas coming out of the common gas outlet of an anaesthetic machine?
Schrader valve on pipeline
Non Interchangeable Screw Thread (NIST) on pipelines
Pin Index identification of cylinders
Colour coding of pipelines, cylinders and connections

HAZARDS

Microshock

1 What order of magnitude of current passing along an intravenous catheter in contact with the myocardium, as shown here (E), is required to induce ventricular fibrillation?
MICROAMPS (absolute value not required)

2 If all this equipment is functioning normally and the patient is not touching metal on the operating table, why is there no risk of microshock?
No direct pathway from patient to earth

3 Are the absolute values of the earth potential relative to the mains at points B, C and D the same?
NO

4 The absolute values of the earth potential relative to the mains of 240 volts may vary. By how much?
Up to two volts

5 How could the absolute values of the earth potential at points B, C and D be made equal (equipotential)?
By connecting points B, C and D to the same physical point

6 If a fault developed in the ECG machine resulting in the patient leads being connected to earth, would microelectrocution (microshock) be more or less likely?
More likely

7 The symbol G may also be found on electrical equipment in theatre. What does it mean?
Equipotential Earth Point

8 The symbol A may also be found on electrical equipment in theatre. What does it mean?
Attention! Read Instructions

9 From this chart (chart 2) identify the meaning of ANY two other symbols.

HISTORY

Varicose veins/asthma

Marks awarded for:

1 *Veins to be stripped on the front and sides only*
2 *Symptoms from the varicose veins (eczema)*
3 *No previous surgery*
4 *Childhood dental GA*
5 *Asthma since teens*
6 *Medication – inhalers (both)*
7 *No systemic steroids*
8 *Exacerbation by chest infection*
9 *Medication – antibiotics*
10 *Influenza vaccine*
11 *Allergies: Must name two of: feathers, fur, cats, house dust*
12 *Allergies proven on skin testing*
13 *Propranolol precipitated major asthma attack*
14 *Other atopy – life long eczema*
15 *Children have hay fever*
16 *Aspirin also precipitates wheezing*

MEASUREMENT

pH

1 Which diagram best represents the hydrogen ion or pH electrode?
Diagram B

2 Assuming diagram B is of a pH electrode, what are the items 'A' made of?
Ag/AgCl

3 Why is it necessary to have two electrodes?
One active and one reference

4 'B' is the reference electrode, what is the solution?
Saturated KCl

5 What is the solution in 'C'?
Buffer

6 What is the item marked 'D'?
H^+ *sensitive glass*

7 What connects the two electrodes?
The blood sample
An electrical circuit

8 The display 'E' reads pH or H^+ concentration, what does it actually measure?
The potential difference between the two electrodes

9 The pH electrode is an integral part of the apparatus for measuring which other physiological parameter?
PCO_2

10 The principle of this electrode can be applied to what other measurements?
Sodium
Potassium
Calcium

11 What chemical equation describes the development of an acidosis by CO_2 accumulation?
$H_2O + CO_2 <-> H_2CO_3 <-> H^+ + HCO_3-$

OSCE Answers

MONITORING

Pulse oximeter

1 Suggest two pieces of information this device provides?
Pulse rate and oxygen saturation

2 In a normal individual, what is the approximate arterial $p0_2$ at point A in graph 1?
8kPa or 60mmHg

3 What name is used to describe point B on graph 1?
p50

4 What use is made of the value of the p50?
Quantifies the movement of the curve left or right in response to influencing factors.

5 What other oxygen-carrying compound has a dissociation curve as shown in graph 2?
Myoglobin

6 What are the wavelengths of the light emitted from the diodes commonly used in pulse oximeters?
660 nm and 940 nm

7 How often do the diodes flash?
Approximately 30 times per second

8 In graph 3, what term is used to describe point A?
Isobestic point

9 If you measured the absorption at point A, what parameter would this reflect?
Total haemoglobin concentration

10 How does a pulse oximeter differentiate between arterial, venous and tissue oxygen saturation?
Calculates only the difference in absorption of the pulsatile flow.

11 Suggest two clinical situations in which a pulse oximeter may be inaccurate?
Peripheral vasoconstriction; hypotension; carbon monoxide poisoning; haemoglobinopathies; arrhythmia; nail varnish; extraneous light; abnormal pigments. (1 mark each for any 2 from list)

12 Suggest a common cause for a pulse oximeter tracing such as in Trace 5?
BP cuff on same arm being inflated and deflated

13 What is the main difference between a clinically used pulse oximeter and a laboratory oximeter which allows the laboratory to report levels of carboxyhaemoglobin and other haemoglobins?
A laboratory oximeter measures absorption at several different wavelengths

PHYSICAL EXAMINATION

Cranial nerves

Marks awarded for performing the following correctly:

1 *Courteous introduction to patient, establishing rapport*

2 *III – Pupillary reactions*

3 *III, IV, VI – Eye movements*

4 *V – Sensation: 3 areas / Motor: mastication or jaw jerk*

5 *VII - Facial movements: raise eyebrows / show teeth*

6 *VIII - Auditory: spoken word / tuning fork*
(vestibular testing not required)

7 *IX – Pharyngeal reflex (description only required)*

8 *X – Vocalisation: say "Ah" and observe movement of soft palate*

9 *XI – Shrug shoulders against resistance*

10 *XII – Protrusion of tongue, inspection for wasting and fasciculation*

11 *Does all of the above in a fluent and co-ordinated manner*

OSCE **Answers**

X-RAY

Cervical spine injury

1 All essential disc spaces are visible
False

2 The anterior longitudinal ligament is undamaged
False

3 The shadow at the tip of 'A' is an abnormality
False

4 There is a fracture of the 2nd cervical vertebra
True

5 This neck will be stable in flexion
False

6 This patient may become apnoeic
True

7 He may develop severe retro-pharyngeal swelling
True

8 Urgent intubation is essential
False

9 Rapid transfer by 'Blue Light' ambulance to a neurosurgical unit is essential
False

10 High dose steroids should be given in casualty
True

RESUSCITATION

Pulseless electrical activity

1 What would you first need to confirm?
There are no signs of life. (Accept patient is in cardiac arrest).

2 An ECG rhythm strip has been recorded. In the absence of a pulse, what is the diagnosis?
Pulseless electrical activity (PEA). [Accept electromechanical dissociation (EMD).]

3 Assuming that the rhythm displayed continues to be slow PEA, how would you proceed?
Recommence CPR at 30:2 for two minutes – check rhythm every two minutes.
Give adrenaline (epinephrine) 1mg IV.
Secure the airway (ETT, LMA) – then continue compressions at 100-120 per minute without pause.

4 What drugs should subsequently be given. How often should the doses be repeated?
Give adrenaline (epinephrine) 1mg intravenously
Repeat every 3-5 minutes (alternate cycles).

5 What reversible factors may be contributing to the failure of this patient to respond?
4 H's (hypoxia, hypovolaemia, hyper/hypokalaemia, hypothermia)
4 T's (tension pneumothorax, tamponade, toxic substances, thromboembolism)

6 In this patient (who is two hours post-op) which of these reversible factors is most likely to be causing this clinical picture?
Hypovolaemia.

7 If the patient responds to fluid resuscitation with the return of a weak pulse, what further actions should you take?
Gain more IV access (minimum of two large-bore cannulae) and give further rapid fluid infusion.
Send blood for cross matching.
Arrange for an urgent laparotomy to control the haemorrhage.

SIM MAN

Endobronchial intubation

Marks awarded for the following:

1 *Comments on abnormal vital signs*

2 *Feels for trachea*

3 *Percusses the chest*

4 *Auscultates the chest and notes reduced air entry*

5 What is the differential diagnosis? (Show blood gas results)
Endobronchial intubation
Worsening gas exchange from aspiration
Pneumonia or other cause of shunting

6 What is the most likely cause for his desaturation?
Endobronchial intubation

7 What is your immediate management?
Candidate should withdraw ETT by about 4 cm
Candidate should auscultate chest to recheck ventilation

8 What other therapeutic manoeuvres may be necessary?
Hand bagging to re-expand the collapsed lung
PEEP

9 What other investigations would be useful?
Chest X-ray
Repeat blood gases

10 Why did the patient not respond to 100% oxygen?
Large shunt (>60%)

TECHNICAL SKILLS

Tracheostomy/Tube change

1 There are a number of important preparations that you should make before attempting the tube change. Describe four of them (accept any four of these)
Stop any enteral feed
Aspirate the nasogastric tube
Put patient on 100% oxygen
Prepare equipment and drugs for orotracheal intubation
Check previous laryngoscopy grade
Suck out trachea and pharynx

2 Having completed your preparations demonstrate how you would carry out the tube change with the equipment provided (i.e. without bougie/guide wire)
Tests cuff in new tube
Deflates cuff and removes existing tube
Inserts new tube with obturator in place
Removes obturator
Inflates cuff in new tube

3 What pressure should you inflate the cuff to?
20-25 cm water

4 At what level should a tracheostomy be sited?
Between 1st and 2nd or 2nd and 3rd tracheal rings

5 A tracheostomy bypasses the upper airway. What functions does the upper airway perform?
Warming
Humidifying
Filtering dust and micro-organisms

6 By what volume does a tracheostomy reduce anatomical deadspace in an adult?
75-100ml (i.e. reduces it to 50-75 ml)

7 In addition to regular suctioning how can we prevent blockage of a tracheostomy tube?
Ensure adequate humidification
Use a double cannula tube with inner tube

8 What type of tracheostomy tube is this?
Variable flange

9 When might you use a variable flange tracheostomy tube?
In an obese patient or if the anatomy is unusual

SOE 1 answers

Pharmacology

Paper 1

Draw a table to compare the physical properties of isoflurane and sevoflurane.

This question is looking for an understanding of how the physical properties of volatile agents affect their clinical properties. Candidates need to know the values for at least boiling point, blood gas partition coefficient and oil gas for sevoflurane, isoflurane and desflurane. In addition, they should be clear as to how these properties affect potency, onset and offset times.

Metabolism of these drugs produces fluoride ions; the potential and clinical importance of this should be understood.

What are the effects of age on renal drug elimination?

Renal function, notably glomerular filtration rate, decreases with age. The question looks at understanding of how this affects elimination of drugs from the body. You should be able to give examples of drugs, where elimination may be significantly affected, e.g. morphine and vecuronium.

How are anti-arrhythmic drugs classified?

They may be classified in several ways but usually using the Vaughan-Williams Classification. This groups drugs according to their effects on the cardiac myocyte action potential. There are four groups with group I having three subgroups. Amiodarone is interesting because it has actions related to several of the classes of anti-arrhythmic drugs.

PAPER 2

What class of drug is vecuronium?

This question is assessing your knowledge and understanding of non-depolarising neuromuscular blocking drugs. You need to demonstrate a clear understanding of their mechanism of action, including being able to explain observations such as fade clearly. You also need to understand the inverse relationship between potency and onset of neuromuscular blockade.

How may drug interactions be classified?

Drugs can interact in many ways. This question is looking at your understanding of the potential interactions of the drugs you use. Pharmacokinetic interactions can affect absorption, distribution, protein binding, metabolism and excretion. You should be able to give examples relevant to your anaesthetic and critical care practice.

What drugs are recommended by NICE for the initial treatment of Type II diabetes mellitus?

Metformin and glicazides. Note other newer agents are not first line treatment, but you will be expected to know what they are. You should be able to explain how metformin and glicazides work, their potential side effects and how they should be managed peri-operatively.

Paper 3

How are opioid receptors classified?

This question is assessing your knowledge of both opioid receptors and receptor theory in general. You should be familiar with the receptor types e.g. MOP, DOP etc. and understand that they are G-protein receptors. You should be able to explain how the G-protein works. In addition, knowledge of the effects of opioids at each receptor would be expected.

Draw a graph of plasma concentration against time following intravenous injection of a drug. (Assume the drug is only distributed in one compartment.)

This question is looking at your understanding of elimination of drugs and the mathematical concepts used to describe this. You should be able to draw the graph of concentration versus time and also its semi-log derivative. Furthermore, you should be able to use these graphs to clearly explain the terms half-life, clearance and volume of distribution and how they can be calculated.

Where in the nephron do diuretic drugs act?

A good way to answer this question is to draw a schematic nephron and use it to show where common diuretic drugs e.g. thiazides, loop diuretics, osmotic agents and acetazolamide work. You will also need a good grasp of the physiology of the kidney to explain how loop diuretics such as frusemide exert their diuretic effect and cause hypokalaemia.

PAPER 4

What is ketamine?

This is a very straightforward question. You will be expected to know what sort of compound ketamine is and how it produces anaesthesia. You should also have a good knowledge of its non-anaesthetic effects notably the cardiovascular, respiratory and neurological. You should also be able to discuss the isomers of ketamine.

Where does drug metabolism take place?

This question is designed to assess your understanding of drug metabolism. It does not look at how a particular drug is metabolised but rather looks for knowledge of the general principles. You should know what the chemical purpose of metabolism is and where metabolism takes place including sites outside the liver. You should be able to explain hepatic drug metabolism including the cytochrome P450 system in some detail.

How do phenothiazines act as anti-emetics?

This is a question where a good diagram of the physiology of nausea and vomiting i.e. vomiting centre and chemoreceptor trigger zone, along with peripheral sites involved, can be invaluable. Such a diagram allows you to quickly and clearly show the examiners how phenothiazines and any other anti-emetic exert their effects.

Note that whilst cyclizine is antihistamine, its anti-emetic effects are thought to be mediated by an effect at cholinergic receptors.

Paper 5

What factors contribute to the onset of inhalational anaesthesia?
This question in common with many will be better answered if you have a structure to hang information off. Here, a simple structure would be to talk about patient factors e.g. minute ventilation and cardiac output and drug factors e.g. blood gas coefficient. Answering in this way rather than offering apparently random factors will help to convey to the examiners that you really understand how inhalational anaesthetics work. You should have a good grasp of the physical properties of inhalational agents that affect their clinical profile.

What is an isomer?
This is a straightforward question again. You should be able to list the different types of isomerism and give examples relevant to anaesthetic practice for each. You should understand how isomers could have very different properties and the clinical usage of this.

What conditions are treated with carbamazepine?
This is a question largely about anti-epileptics but you should be aware of the other clinical indications for carbamazepine. You need to be able to classify the anti-epileptics according to mode of action and place carbamazepine in the appropriate group.

Paper 6

What drugs can be used to reverse neuromuscular blockade?

This question is primarily assessing your knowledge of anti-cholinesterase. In addition to neostigmine you should also be aware of short-acting and long-acting anti-cholinesterases as well as the organo-phosphorus poisons. You should be able to relate their activity to their molecular chemistry. You should also have a clear idea of the non-neuromuscular effects of acetylcholine and how these may be reduced in clinical practice.

How can receptors be classified?

This question assesses your understanding of receptor theory. You should know the common receptor types in the human body e.g. ion channels, G-protein linked and steroid. You will need to be able to discuss these receptors with reference to response time and magnification of response. You should be able to describe the G-protein, including its subtypes in detail with examples of ligands.

What is co-amoxiclav?

This question is assessing your understanding of antibiotic resistance. You need to demonstrate an understanding of the mechanisms by which bacteria can exhibit resistance and how resistance can spread. You should be able to discuss clearly mechanisms of reducing resistance. It may be useful to classify these, for example into general measures and pharmacological measures.

Paper 7

What is the site of action of benzodiazepines?

This is a relatively straightforward test of knowledge. However, you must be able to explain exactly how benzodiazepines exert their effect on the $GABA_A$ receptor. You will need to understand clearly how the $GABA_A$ receptor works. You will also need to demonstrate that you know the indications for benzodiazepines and how to administer them safely.

Draw a dose response curve for a full agonist.

This question looks at your understanding of receptor ligand interactions. You need to able to draw both a dose response curve and a log-dose response and explain the advantages of one over the other. You then need to use these curves to explain terms including: potency, affinity, efficacy, partial agonism, and competitive and non-competitive antagonism. You should practise drawing these curves during your revision.

Where are Histamine Type 1 receptors found in the human body?

This is a factual question. You should know where histamine receptors are located and the effects of histamine on them. You should be able to discuss the difference between first generation antihistamines and later generations in terms of their side effect profiles.

Paper 8

Describe the mechanism of action of local anaesthetics?

The key to this question is an understanding of how local anaesthetics work. You need to know that they are weak bases and what this actually means. You need to be able to clearly discuss the term pKa and use this to explain onset. This also requires a good understanding of their action on nerve ion channels. You should be able to discuss other properties of local anaesthetics such as length of action and show an understanding of how their chemistry and handling by the body may affect this.

What are the causes of inter-patient variability to drugs?

This is a question that lends itself to being answered with a sound structure. The natural tendency is to leap into genetics forgetting that there are other causes of inter-patient variability e.g. age, race, disease states etc. It is important to discuss these in a full answer. You will need to be able to explain how genetics may affect drug response with relevant examples.

Which drugs can be used to reduce stomach acidity?

To answer this question requires a grasp of the physiology of acid production. It lends itself to the use of a diagram of the parietal cell showing the stages in production and regulation of gastric acid. This can be used to clearly demonstrate where the various drug groups used to reduce acidity exert their effects.

PAPER 9

Compare the non-anaesthetic effects of isoflurane and desflurane.

A good structure is fundamental to answering this question well. The question lends itself to a body systems approach, i.e. cardiovascular, respiratory, renal, endocrine etc. A thorough knowledge of the cardiovascular effects will be particularly important.

What types of data can be seen in medical research?

It is important to know that statistics can be examined as part of the pharmacology SOE. The questions are generally straightforward and fact based.

You should know the common types of data e.g. continuous, non-, continuous, categorical, ordinal etc. and how to graphically demonstrate such data. You need to know the difference between parametric and non-parametric data and know tests that are suitable for both types.

How can drugs affect platelet function?

In common with many general pharmacology questions this one requires an understanding of platelet and clotting physiology. Once again a diagram of a platelet clearly showing the receptors that are activated during platelet aggregation and adhesion, is an excellent way to answer this question. You then need to show clearly where the various anti-platelet agents exert their effects.

You should be familiar with guidelines concerning surgery, anaesthesia and the common anti-platelet agents.

Paper 10

What is aspirin?

The key to this question is a thorough understanding of the arachidonic acid pathway, cyclo-oxygenase and their role in the production of prostaglandins. You should then be able to demonstrate where aspirin acts and the implications of this both in terms of pain relief and the side effects of aspirin.

Which esterases are relevant to anaesthetic practice?

This question is largely about plasma cholinesterase but you should be aware of other cholinesterases and where in the body they are found e.g. red blood cells.

You need to understand how disease both acquired and hereditary can affect plasma cholinesterase function. You will need to be able to discuss suxamethonium apnoea in some detail including the genetic variants.

How are red cells prepared and stored for transfusion?

This is a straightforward factual question. You should be able to discuss what is in a bag of red cells and what is not, relative to whole blood. You should know the storage constituents and what the purpose of each one is. You should know where and how blood is stored in your hospital. You will need to have a thorough understanding of the hazards of blood transfusion.

Physiology answers

Paper 1

Identify the abnormalities in these arterial blood gases: pH 7.03, $PaCO_2$ 7.3 kPa, PaO_2 7.1 kPa

Define pH, and relate to normal values.

What additional information may assist interpretation? Include discussion of standard bicarbonate, base excess and anion gap.

Discuss effect on pH of chronic hypercapnia.

What are the mechanisms of metabolic compensation? You will be expected to describe these in detail and discuss how they change with time.

If you are given any question on arterial blood gases you will be expected to discuss how the values are inter-related and give a reasoned response as to the likely cause(s).

Describe the anatomical organisation of the pituitary gland

Anterior – portal hypophyseal circulation. Posterior – neurones from hypothalamus.

Contrast the control of posterior and anterior pituitary hormone release: Anterior – hypophysiotropic hormones via portal circulation. Posterior – neurones from hypothalamus.

What is the effect of ADH release on the body? Osmotic pressure changes, extracellular fluid volume, stress, nausea, alcohol.

Endocrine questions will require you to be able to explain the different feedback and control mechanisms involved.

What determines the membrane potential of a nerve fibre?

Explain differences between Nernst equation and Goldman equation and how they relate to the ion concentrations inside and outside the neurone.

What are the important differences between peripheral nerve and cardiac muscle action potentials? Use diagrams to illustrate your answer. Discuss origin of impulse, plateau phase and tetany. Mode of conduction.

Paper 2

Draw a diagram to show the relationship between cerebral blood flow and blood pressure

Discuss cerebral blood flow, mean arterial pressure and autoregulation, effects of hypertension etc.

What are the theories of the mechanism of cerebral autoregulation? Metabolic (local), myogenic, neural.

Discuss the effect of changes in PO_2, PCO_2 on cerebral blood flow and intracranial pressure. Graphs should be used to demonstrate the principles involved.

Effects of anaesthesia on cerebral blood flow and cerebral oxygen uptake.

What types of immunity are there?

Non-specific - barrier mechanisms, local inflamm responses (lysozyme, complement, NK cells). Specific – T and B cell mechanisms.

What type of hypersensitivity reactions do you know? Four types: 1 – allergic igE, 2 – ab dependent cytotoxic, 3 – immune complex mediated, 4 – cell mediated delayed. Give example of each.

Although this question may appear difficult, a good structure to your answer will help you to develop your answer and draw on your knowledge.

What is the respiratory response to rebreathing 5% CO_2 in oxygen?

Draw the response in a spontaneously breathing subject. Linear relationship (CO_2 response curve)

What is the response to breathing a hypoxic mixture? Rectangular hyperbola.

Explain the diagrams in detail including the mechanisms of the response via central and peripheral chemoreceptors.

Paper 3

Define hypoxia

Definition and classification of causes. Discuss types – hypoxic, anaemic, stagnant and histotoxic.

Draw an oxy-haemoglobin dissociation curve for saturation showing arterial and mixed venous points in the four types of hypoxia.

What is oxygen content?

Discuss arterial and venous oxygen content values in each of the four types of hypoxia.

In the kidney, how is glomerular filtrate produced?

Explain physiological process of filtration and factors affecting filtration rate.

How and why is inulin used to assess renal function? Discuss alternatives along with their limitations

How does the body respond to changes in systemic blood pressure?

Changes in vascular resistance and cardiac output to compensate.

Discuss physiological changes associated with change in preload compared with change in afterload.

Explain the role of the low- and high-pressure baroreceptors, and the renin–angiotensin–aldosterone system.

Paper 4

How is oxygen transported from the lungs to the cells of the tissues?

Role of red blood cell. Diffusion across alveolus to pulmonary capillary; oxygen carriage by blood; diffusion from capillary to mitochondria.

What is the oxygen content of the blood? Give arterial and mixed venous values and show how these values are derived.

What methods can be used to increase oxygen content and oxygen. delivery? Use the equation to guide your answer.

What function does vomiting serve?

Protective reflex pathway. Chemoreceptor trigger zone (CTZ), vomiting centre.

Afferent inputs, diagram of inter-connections.

Role of dopamine, acetylcholine, histamine, serotonin. Hypotension.

CTZ and blood–brain barrier.

What physiological changes occur during vomiting? Take it system by system i.e. GI, respiratory, cardiovascular.

Explain the events in the cardiac cycle

You may be given a diagram so start at one place and explain the events. Annotate the diagram with values and show where valves open and close.

Superimpose aortic and left atrial pressures.

What general factors affect cardiac output? Rate, stroke volume, myocardial contractility. Starling curves, dP/dt.

Paper 5

Define ventilation perfusion (V/Q) ratio

Definition, normal value and range.

What variation of ventilation and perfusion occurs within the lung? Discuss changes of each from apex to base with reasons.

Discuss effects of high and low V/Q on alveolar O_2 and CO_2 partial pressures.

Contrast the sympathetic and parasympathetic nervous systems

Outflow – craniosacral/thoracolumbar, neurotransmitters in ganglia and end organs.

Acetylcholine nicotinic, muscarinic. Catecholaminergic, sympathetic cholinergic etc.

Comparative effects on body organs.

Heart/circulation, digestive system/skin.

Describe the factors controlling the movement of fluid across the pulmonary capillary walls

Starling forces, oncotic and hydrostatic pressure changes along the pulmonary capillary. Permeability and reflection coefficients.

Compare with systemic capillary.

Describe lymphatic drainage.

What role does the pulmonary vascular endothelium have?

Vascular control, metabolism, anticoagulant.

Paper 6

How is CO_2 transported from the cells to the lungs?

Carbamino-compounds, bicarbonate, dissolved. You need to know the proportion of each and details of how they influence carbon dioxide carriage.

Discuss the events in the plasma/RBC. Carbonic anhydrase – role.

What are the important properties of the bicarbonate buffer system? pKa, abundance, open system.

Using a straight line to represent the length of the convoluted tubule from Bowman's capsule to the start of the Loop of Henle, show the concentrations of glucose, sodium and inulin (assuming using it to measure GFR)

Explain diagram and the physiology in detail – values will depend on whether substances are reabsorbed or secreted and may be influenced by movement of other solutes.

What are the transport mechanisms involved? Passive and active processes, thresholds and limits.

How much glucose is filtered by the kidney?

What physiological factors increase GFR? Starling's forces; membrane permeability; afferent/efferent arterioles.

How does release of acetylcholine from an alpha motor neurone lead to muscle contraction?

Describe the process.

Neuromuscular junction, neurotransmission, MEPPs, action potential, cholinesterases.

Mechanism of muscle contraction. Role of calcium, t tubules, actin, myosin, sarcolemma.

Paper 7

Draw an action potential for a sinoatrial node cell

Draw the diagram with labelled axes and indicate the phases; relate to ion fluxes.

Mechanism of spontaneous depolarisation.

Effect of vagal stimulation; sympathetic stimulation on the action potential and relate to changes in heart rate.

What receptors are involved? Ach, G proteins etc.

How does neonatal physiology differ from adult physiology?

Discuss respiratory differences, compliance, surfactant, HbF.

Cardiovascular, body fluid compartments and blood volume?

Renal, hepatic: sodium, fluid and drug handling.

Discuss heat losses and their control in the neonate.

What would happen if you trod on a pin in your bare feet?

Describe reflex. Afferents, reflex pathway, nerve fibre size, conduction velocity, cell bodies, efferents.

What happens in the contralateral limb? (the other leg)

Contrast with the stretch reflex: polysynaptic vs. monosynaptic reflexes.

What are the functions of these reflexes? Protective mechanisms.

Paper 8

What is the relationship between BP, SVR and CO?

Relate to Ohm's Law.

Describe the reflexes elicited by a rapid fall in blood pressure. Firing of the baroreceptors and feedback loop.

What is the role of low-pressure baroreceptors? Location and function.

Describe the role of the renin–angiotensin–aldosterone system. Include medium-term control of blood pressure. Time course.

What are the body's basic metabolic requirements for exercise?

Oxygen and energy source.

What are the muscle energy sources and their duration during **aerobic** exercise? Initially ATP/creatine-phophate, then glycogen and fats.

What is oxygen deficit/oxygen debt? Draw a diagram of VO_2/exercise time

You will need to know about the anaerobic threshold and differences between aerobic and anaerobic metabolism.

How can the partial pressure of oxygen in alveolar gas be calculated?

Explain how PiO_2 is calculated.

Use alveolar gas equation to discuss effect of atmospheric pressure, saturated vapour pressure, H_2O etc.

What factors affect the RQ – diet.

Discuss metabolism of different food substrates, carbohydrates, fats proteins etc.

Draw a curve to demonstrate the effect of changes in minute ventilation on PAO_2.

Add the curve for CO_2.

Paper 9

Describe the physiological responses to the rapid IV infusion of 1 L of normal saline

Distribution between compartments. Intracellular, extracellular, interstitial and barriers between. Low- high-pressure baroreceptors.

Low pressure: atria and atrial natriuretic peptide

High pressure: baroreceptor reflex.

Effect on the kidneys of reduced aldosterone.

How does the body handle a glucose load?

Beta-cell secretion, from precursor molecule. Decreases plasma glucose by increasing uptake into cells and promoting anabolic pathways.

Describe the metabolism of glucose. Energy production (glycolysis, TCA cycle, etc); glycogen production; conversion to fat/proteins.

How is glucose handled by the kidney? Discuss tubular reabsorption in detail with mechanisms.

During mechanical ventilation what is the effect on $PaCO_2$ of altering minute ventilation?

Draw a graph to aid your explanation.

What are the physiological effects of altering $PaCO_2$? Give your answer systematically – cardiovascular, CNS, renal etc.

What is the effect on PaO_2 of altering minute ventilation? Use a graph to explain.

Think about your answer and listen carefully to the question as it is easy to confuse the effects of altering minute ventilation on arterial blood gas values and the effect of changes in PaO_2 and $PaCO_2$ on minute ventilation.

Paper 10

On a diagram showing a normal ECG trace for two cardiac cycles draw left ventricular pressure changes first and then aortic pressure changes on the same time axis

Explain waveforms.

What is isovolumetric contraction? Where do the valves open?

Demonstrate an understanding of events with timescales.

What is mean arterial pressure? Indicate on diagram.

Describe the metabolic response to starvation

Overview of glycogenolysis, gluconeogenesis, muscle catabolism.

What is the endocrine control of the metabolic response?

Insulin, glucagon, cortisol, epinephrine (adrenaline) actions.

Describe the receptor/intracellular mechanisms that bring about these changes.

Receptors involved, mechanisms of action etc. Protein changes.

Which organs are involved in gluconeogenesis? Liver, kidney.

Describe the structure of a skeletal muscle fibre. Myofibrils, sarcomere as basic unit. Striations: A, I & H bands; Z- and M-lines

How and why do cardiac and skeletal muscle differ? Functional anatomy; electrophysiology, receptors (Ach nicotinic and muscarinic, adrenergic etc.)

Explain mechanism of excitation – contraction. Cellular biochemical events in detail.

Tina McLeod

SOE 2 answers

Clinical anaesthesia

Paper 1

Airway assessment/difficult intubation

A healthy 35-year-old woman is on your list for an elective laparoscopic cholecystectomy and you find that she can only open her mouth by two fingers' breadth. What further information would you like to know?

History (difficult intubation)

- Previous GAs (get records), pre-disposing trauma/surgery/disease (rheumatoid, scleroderma, etc.)
- Examination (re: difficult intubation)
- Anatomical features associated with difficult intubation.
- Mallampati, thyro-mental distance, malocclusion, atlanto-occipital distance, etc.

Anaesthetic plan

- GA: LMA *vs* TT. The role of inhalational induction to assess airway Fibreoptic intubation (awake *vs* GA?)
- Senior help. Grades of laryngoscopy (I–IV)
- Information to patient later
- Emphasis on diagnosis, recognition and safe management of a difficult airway

Laryngospasm

At the end of the procedure the patient is extubated. Immediately thereafter, she develops severe laryngospasm. How will you assess and manage this situation?

Diagnostic signs

- Complete obstruction: obstructive 'see-saw' movements of chest and abdomen, tracheal tug, oxygen desaturation, signs of hypercarbia, extreme patient anxiety (if conscious), may show signs of incomplete reversal of neuromuscular block
- Partial obstruction: all of above with stridor

Management

- Summon help, clear action plan always ensuring oxygenation

Post-operative nausea and vomiting

Are patients liable to post-operative nausea and vomiting (PONV) after cholecystectomy?

(Occurrence and prevention of PONV)

Predisposition

- Young age, women, anxiety, obesity, history of motion sickness, hypoxia, hypotension, history of PONV
- Gynaecological, middle ear surgery, gut distension. Role of opioids, volatiles, N_2O

Prevention

- Pre-op visit, anti-emetic premedication, reduction of gastric stasis, use of anxiolytics. Use of anaesthetic techniques: TIVA, regional anaesthesia, avoidance of opioids

Treatment (clinical aspects of PONV)

- Use of multiple anti-emetics, avoidance of opioids, treat pain, prevent gastric stasis, rehydration

Paper 2

Ten-year-old child presenting for tonsillectomy

A ten-year-old boy presents for elective tonsillectomy. The indication for surgery is excessive snoring and disturbed sleep. He has a history of asthma and takes regular beclometasone diproprionate (Becotide) but is otherwise healthy. He had a cold one week ago, but his parents say he is now fully recovered.

How would you assess this child pre-operatively?

Presenting complaint

- Snoring (obstructive sleep apnoea?), last episode of tonsillitis, urgency of surgery?

Asthma

- Assess severity: frequency, admissions, Causative factors (e.g. URTI), other medication, NSAIDs

Implications of recent 'cold'

- URTI totally resolved
- Increase in peri-op complications, e.g. laryngospasm, hypoxia, bronchospasm
- Criteria for cancellation of child with recent URTI

General assessment

- Weight height, airway, teeth, veins, co-operation!
- Past anaesthetic history/family history/allergy

Anaesthetic plan

What is your anaesthetic plan for this child?

Consent

Fasting guidelines

Premedication

- Sedative (dose, onset time), EMLA, Ametop (onset time)

Intra-op

- Parents in anaesthetic room?
- TT *vs* LMA (sizes) IPPV vs SV (circuit)
- Induction: IV or inhalation (technique, drugs, doses)
- Maintenance, analgesia, anti-emetic (doses), fluids
- Awake or deep extubation (pros and cons)

Post-operative care

After handing over the care of the boy to the recovery staff, you are called back because he is extremely distressed. What might be the cause? (post-operative care: analgesia and other issues)

Cause of distress

- Pain
- Bleeding
- Nausea, vomiting
- Anxiety, absence of parents

Post-operative analgesia

- Potent analgesia in recovery (what, how)
- Paracetamol/NSAID (dose/route/cautions)
- Other options: oral morphine regime
- Pain assessment in children

Other post-operative care

- Anti-emesis, fluid management

Paper 3

Elective RIH repair in a 46-year-old with diabetes

A 46-year-old male, (who has had Type 1 diabetes since the age of 14), has been admitted for repair of a right-sided inguinal hernia. When you meet him he has a normal BP, HR and temperature. He takes atenolol. What important things would you be looking for at the pre-operative visit?

Main problems

- Diabetes
- Treated hypertension

Diabetes:

- Insulin regimen and control: glycosylated haemoglobin levels
- Co-morbidities; cardiac, renal, microvascular
- Peri-operative management

Hypertension

- Relevance to anaesthesia
- Effectiveness of therapy
- Assessment of end organ damage

Peri-operative management

- Position on operating list
- GA versus regional versus local
- Performing a spinal block: methods, complications etc.
- Intubation: performing difficult intubation, methods
- Management of anaesthesia, drugs chosen etc.
- Assessing when a patient can be extubated

Sudden convulsion in recovery

This patient is transferred to the Post Anaesthetic Care Area and shortly afterwards suffers a convulsion. What will you do?

Differential diagnosis

- Hypoglycaemia, hyponatraemia, sepsis, CVA, pre-existing epilepsy

Management of convulsion

- ABC + drugs

Where will post-operative care best be carried out?

- General ward, HDU, ITU?

Management of concurrent medication

What regular medication taken by a patient would you ensure was taken on the day of surgery?

Diabetes

- Oral agents, insulin

CVS

- Therapy for hypertension, angina, arrhythmias

Anti-coagulants

- Warfarin, heparins, anti-platelet agents

Respiratory

- Inhalers, oral steroids (peri-op cover)

Psychiatric

- Lithium, MAO

Analgesics

- Chronic use, fentanyl patch, opioid abusers

Paper 4

Unrousable 29-year-old emergency admission

You are called to the A&E Department at midnight to attend an 'unrousable' 29-year-old man who has been brought in by his friends from a party where he had collapsed. His breathing is irregular and laboured.

How will you proceed?

ABC (expand)

- Conscious level assessment: AVPU, Glasgow coma score

Differential diagnosis

- Alcohol, drugs, neurological, metabolic, trauma, haemorrhage, sepsis

Investigations

- Toxicology screen (blood/urine), routine haematology, biochemistry (hyponatraemia), CT scan, LP, blood cultures
- Whole body survey: trauma, sepsis

He develops neurological signs and needs an urgent CT head scan

How will you proceed?

Priorities

- Senior help, airway management (full stomach), RSI, ensure oxygenation and ventilation
- Indications for intubation and ventilation
- GCS < 8, loss of pharyngeal reflexes, hypoventilation, hypoxia, hypercarbia

What precautions would you take to reduce secondary brain injury

- Avoid hypotension, hypercarbia, hypoxia
- Avoid glucose-containing solutions
- Role of mannitol/hypertonic saline

Anaesthesia during scan

- Technique. Remote site, transfer issues, problem of access in scanner

Needle stick injury

During your management of this case you suffer a needle stick injury with a needle contaminated with this patient's blood. What action would you take?

Contamination reduction

- Wash, promote bleeding. Do not suck or scrub

Assess risk with HIV. Hep B, Hep C

- Seroconversion rates 0.5%, 20%, ≈5% respectively

Post exposure prophylaxis and counselling

- Take blood from patient and self to confirm status (consent issues) and report injury
- Hep B: immunoglobulin and vaccination (vaccination status)
- Hep C: no post-exposure prophylaxis available
- HIV: combination ante-retroviral therapy ASAP

Other infection transmission risks during surgery

- Prions, TB, compromised patients: MRSA

Preventative measures

- Disposable equipment, filters, facemasks

Paper 5

Assessment of trauma and multiple injuries

You are called to the accident and emergency department to assist with the care of a 17-year-old who has crashed his motorcycle. He has multiple injuries.

What are the priorities in your resuscitation of this patient?

- ABC of resuscitation
- Immediate care of cervical spine; cervical stabilisation and care with intubation
- Diagnosis and treatment of pneumothorax/haemothorax
- Primary and secondary survey
- Priorities in management
- Diagnosis and management of hypovolaemic shock, assessment of blood loss
- Fluid types and volumes requirement for blood transfusion etc.
- Vascular access in trauma patients
- Glasgow coma scale
- Pain management
- Abdominal injuries and late diagnosis
- Requirement for imaging to aid management

Examination reveals a rigid abdomen

How would you anaesthetise this patient?

Anaesthesia for hypovolaemic patient

- RSI – technique and doses
- Monitoring
- Management of hypotension post-induction

Assessment of blood loss and coagulopathy

- Blood and clotting factor replacement

Post-op management

- General ward or critical care
- Analgesia: systemic *vs* regional
- Post-splenectomy issues

Wrong blood

The surgery is proceeding when it is realised that the patient has been given the wrong blood. What problems may the patient develop as a result?

Normal checks when giving blood to patients

Consequences of giving the wrong blood (transfusion reaction)

- Temperature rise
- Wheals near infusion site
- Hypotension
- Anaphylaxis
- Haemolysis
- DIC

How would you manage a case of wrong blood transfusion?

- Stop transfusion, supportive therapy

What are the other problems with blood transfusion?

- Immune problems
- Infection risk: Hep A, B, C, non A/non B, HIV, CMV, CJD
- Massive transfusion: hypervolaemia, dilution problems, hyperkalaemia, hypocalcaemia, hypothermia, TRALI

Paper 6

Hypertensive for hernia repair

You are asked to anaesthetise an obese 54-year-old patient for elective hernia repair. He has hypertension controlled by diuretic medication, but on admission to the ward a nurse records his BP as 165/105 mm Hg. Would you postpone elective surgery with such an admission BP?

Hypertension

- Significance of one-off BP measurement
- Accuracy of BP measurement
- Obesity and hypertension. Obesity: body mass index
- Urgency of procedure
- Hypertension and anaesthesia. Myocardial oxygen demand/supply

Anaesthetic plan (assume BP settles to 155/95 mm Hg)

- RA Vs GA *vs* LA: pros and cons
- RA: spinal *vs* epidural
- LA: infiltration; agent, dose, technique
- GA: tracheal tube *vs* LMA
- Spontaneous respiration *vs* IPPV
- Post-operative analgesia

ST segment changes on ECG

The patient insists on a GA. Halfway through the procedure you notice marked ST segment changes on the ECG. How do you proceed?

Causes

- Myocardial ischaemia (+/- ischaemic heart disease)
- Quickly exclude easily remediable causes: hypoxia, hypotension, brady- or tachy-arrhythmia, hypertension, hypercarbia (hypoventilation, circuit leaks, rebreathing, MH)

Management

- Maximise oxygenation, correct precipitating cause (discuss)
- Summon help, do not proceed with surgery
- Consider GTN patch/infusion, change volatile?
- Lead ECG, Troponin T, check U&Es, acid base status
- If changes transient, continue with surgery?
- Post-operative care?

Pre-operative visiting and premedication

Why do we visit patients pre-operatively on the ward?

Identification of patient. Rapport

Information for patient and anaesthetist (and relatives, e.g. parents of young, children of elderly)

- Discussion of premedication and anaesthetic techniques
- Post-op pain relief: HDU, ICU etc.

Associated medical problems

- Investigation results

Premedication

- Anxiolysis, anti-emesis, drugs, pre emptive analgesia etc. DVT prophylaxis

Consent

- Rectal administration, regional anaesthesia, etc.
- Role of the anaesthetist in ensuring checking consent
- Children

SOE Answers

Paper 7

Emergency laparotomy in an 82-year-old man

A man of 82 years (previously fit and on no medications) presents for emergency laparotomy for presumed perforated bowel. He has passed a total of 100 ml urine over the last 8 hours. He is alert but slightly breathless when speaking. BP=100/60, pulse 105/min.

Is there anything in his history, which you feel, needs more investigation and management prior to surgery?

Oliguria

- Pre-renal, renal, post-renal
- Rehydration and fluid replacement

Breathlessness

- Heart failure or chest infection? – diagnosis and management

CVS

- Assessment, invasive lines, resuscitation (how much time available)

Anaesthetic technique and intra-operative event

Following appropriate resuscitation of this patient, how would you proceed with general anaesthesia?

Anaesthetic technique

- Full stomach, NG tube (stomach empty?)
- Rapid sequence, choice of agents/doses
- Monitoring = invasive
- Epidural for intra- and post-operative use (pros and cons)

Following induction of anaesthesia, there is a profound drop in BP and a fall in $EtCO_2$ associated with high ventilating pressures. What do you do?

Differential diagnosis

- Tension pneumothorax (after CVP), anaphylaxis, ventilator malfunction

Signs and symptoms of tension pneumothorax
Management

- First line treatment – needle thoracocentesis
- Second line – formal chest drain insertion. Site and technique
- High dependency or intensive care

Why might this patient require ventilation on an ITU?

Hypoxia, CVS instability, hypothermia, sepsis, prolonged surgery, metabolic and electrolyte abnormality

Ventilation issues

- Drugs required to facilitate IPPV
- Basic ventilatory modes
- Monitoring of ventilation on ITU

Scoring systems on ITU: description, value, limitations

Paper 8

COPD for hernia repair

A male 76-year-old heavy smoker with severe chronic obstructive pulmonary disease has a right inguinal hernia which is to be repaired electively. He requests a spinal anaesthetic because a friend of his had one recently for a prostatectomy and he thought it would be 'good for his chest'.

Do you think this will be a suitable choice of anaesthetic?

Possible contraindications to spinal anaesthesia

COPD assessment

- History (exercise tolerance, cough, sputum, ankle oedema, orthopnoea, admissions, medication – steroids/home oxygen)
- Examination (demeanour, posture, ability to speak, respiratory rate, accessory muscles, cyanosis, pursed lips, clubbing, auscultation, signs of cor pulmonale
- Investigations (SpO_2 on air, CXR, ABGs, sputum, PFTs)

Pre-operative optimisation

- Physiotherapy, antibiotics, brochodilators etc.
- Urgency of surgery

Anaesthetic technique and complications

How would you establish appropriate spinal anaesthesia for this patient?

Spinal anaesthesia technique

- Height of block required. Use of benzodiazepines/sedation

Post-operative care

- Analgesia, O_2 therapy precautions

Ten minutes after the onset of spinal anaesthesia he becomes very pale and drowsy. What do you do?

Assessment

- ABC: conscious? chest pain/SOB? BP, SpO_2, ECG: rate/rhythm/ST changes
- Block height. Anaphylaxis signs?
- Timing in relation to spinal, other drugs

Differential diagnosis

- Hypotension due to spinal block, high spinal, arrhythmia, MI, anaphylaxis

Management

- Call for help
- Hypotension: fluids. Vasopressors: type?
- Ensure breathing/oxygenation

Post-operative confusion

Twenty four hours later, you are asked to review the patient on the ward. The ward staff say he has been extremely confused and agitated since the operation. Why might this be?

Post-operative confusion

- Often no obvious precipitating cause
- Hypoxia, hypercapnia (chest infection?)
- Hypotension, arrhythmia (¬AF, MI?)
- Electrolyte disturbance (hyponatraemia)
- Pyrexia (chest, UTI, etc.)
- CVA
- Drug effect (opioid, tramadol, cyclizine, etc. Alcohol withdrawal)

Assesment, investigation, management

Paper 9

Obese patient for a hysteroscopy

A 57-year-old lady is listed as a gynaecology day case for a hysteroscopy. You see her on the morning of surgery and discover that she is of average height and weighs 112 kg. She describes recent episodes of chest pain.

What aspects of her history are you interested in?

Obesity

- Define (BMI)
- Associated co-morbidity
- Anaesthetic implications (anatomical, physiological, pharmacological, technical)

Chest pain

- Angina, GORD, musculoskeletal, respiratory
- IHD: assessment, investigate, treat? Anaesthetic implications of IHD

Presenting complaint

- Anaemia? Neoplasia?

Anaesthetic technique

This patient insists on a general anaesthetic. How would you proceed?

Suitability as day case?

Risks of general anaesthesia

Anaesthetic technique

- Pros and cons of LMA *vs* TT (RSI, awake?), IPPV *vs* spont resp
- Calculation of drug doses
- Lithotomy position and its problems: pressure points and damage
- Monitoring: cuff size and BP

Difficulty breathing in recovery

After handing over the care of the patient to the recovery staff, you are called back because she is having difficulty breathing. What might be the cause?

Differential diagnosis

- Upper airway obstruction, bronchospasm (+/- aspiration, anaphylaxis) poor reversal of any NM blockade, atelectasis/lobar collapse, pulmonary embolus, pulmonary oedema (MI?)

Assessment

- ABC
- SaO_2 +/- ABG, CXR, ECG

Management

- Call for help
- Initial: CPAP 100% O_2 (humidified)
- Further: intubate?, supportive care, ITU/HDU

Paper 10

Elective Caesarean section

A 19-year-old primigravida at 39 weeks' gestation is booked for elective Caesarean section because of a transverse presentation.

What are the main anaesthetic issues with such cases?

Care of mother and baby

- General health and health during pregnancy: pre-eclampsia, excess weight gain

Implications of physiology and pharmacology changes of pregnancy

- Aspiration risk, intubation difficulty, CVS/resp changes

Anaesthetic technique

- Regional *vs* GA
- Patient positioning
- Technique for spinal or CSE (LA/adjuncts)
- Block assessment
- Control of blood pressure
- Implications of oxytocin

Difficulty breathing after onset of spinal anaesthesia

You decide to perform a spinal anaesthetic, but after the spinal injection, the patient complains of severe breathing difficulty. What do you do?

Initial management priorities

- High spinal (assess block), +/- anaphylaxis, PE, AFE
- Airway: ensure safe airway and oxygenation: intubation?
- Hypotension control

Decision to proceed with surgery, ensure anaesthesia

Post-operative care

- Higher level care: HDU

Headache

Why might a woman complain of a headache 24 hours after a Caesarean section under spinal anaesthesia?

Causes

- Post-dural puncture (epidural +/- 1%, much less common after spinal)
- Existing condition: migraine, sinusitis. NB – lack of sleep, exhaustion, dehydration, general discomfort
- Cerebro-vascular event (bleed/thrombus)
- Sepsis: CNS or systemic

Management of post-dural puncture headache

Topics to be covered when informing patients of risks of regional anaesthesia?

SOE Answers

Physics and clinical measurement, equipment and safety

Paper 1

Graphical relationships

Show diagrams and ask candidate if they recognise any of them. Go on from there.

- Exponentials:
  - Tear away (bacterial growth)
  - Wash in (drugs, pressure generator)
  - Wash out (drugs, exhalation)
- Properties of exponentials – half-life, time constant
- Effect of log plots
- Straight line: $y = mx+c$, slope is m, c gives intercept
- Direct relationships, e.g. Charles' Law (volume directly proportional to temperature)
- Rectangular hyperbola
- $x.y =$ constant or $y = 1/x$
- Inverse relationships, e.g. Boyle's law, isotherms, $PaCO_2$ and alveolar ventilation

Needles used in anaesthetic practice

Show photograph of Tuohy needle – what is this needle used for? Ask candidate to describe detail of design and relate to function.

- Stillette, cm markings, Huber tip, gauge
- Discuss flow – Poiseuille's formula
- Contrast design with spinal needles
- Safety features

pH Electrodes

What units do we use to measure the acidity of a blood sample?

- Definition of pH
- Relationship between pH and mmol/L of H^+
- Principle of action, ion-specific membrane
- Reference electrode
- Potentiometric electrodes (pH, PCO_2) versus amperometric (PO_2)
- Calibration errors, drift, membrane damage and contamination
- Sampling errors, effect of over-heparinisation; delays in analysis

Paper 2

Electrical circuit components; defibrillation

Show candidate the card with various electrical symbols. Do you recognise any of those symbols on the card? What are they?

- Properties, applications and units etc. of resistor, capacitor, inductor, earth, diode, battery, amplifier, transformer
- Resistor application of Ohm's Law
- Capacitor capacitance of 1 farad holds a charge of 1 coulomb if 1 volt across plates F = C/V: 1 coulomb is charge passing when 1 amp flows for 1 s: C = amp x s
- Inductor inductance of 1 Henry
- Diode rectification; voltage stabilisation (Zener)
- Amplifier voltage from transducers and voltage for recorders
- Transformer: double insulation, step up and step down
- Components of defibrillator: what is the physiological objective; circuit diagram; function of capacitor (to store energy); function of inductor (to control time of discharge); measuring the shock (joules, say 30 amp for 3 ms from 5000 V), energy delivered to patient *vs* stored energy, surface contact, internal and external, synchronised.
- Monophasic versus biphasic: differences and waveforms

Resuscitation bags and valves

What type of resuscitation bag do you find on a cardiac arrest trolley? How does it work?

- Principles and importance of self-inflating bag (photograph)
- Max FiO_2 achievable; on air, with O_2 added to inlet, with addition of bag
- Importance of inspiratory flow in relation to FiO_2 achieved
- Pressure-limiting valves
- Adult and paediatric bags
- Types of valve fitted, e.g. AMBU, Laerdal
- FiO_2 depends on type of valve in use during spontaneous respiration which allows breath from air or from bag contents
- Other equipment found on resuscitation trolley: pre-filled syringes, laryngoscopes, tubes, oesophageal obturators, laryngeal masks, defibrillators

Indirect blood pressure measurement

How do you measure blood pressure on the ward?

- Devices uses and their principles
  - Palpation or auscultation (Korotkoff sounds)
  - Aneroid gauges
  - Mercury manometers
  - Oscillometry (DINAMAP)
  - Penaz technique (Finapres)
- Complications, limitation and errors
  - Cuff size: width 40% mid-circumference of arm and length should be twice width
  - Cuff is accurate at normotension: underestimates hypertension and over-estimates hypotension
  - Bradycardias and arrhythmias
  - Delay in reading
  - Tourniquet effects: nerve damage
- Indications for invasive blood pressure monitoring

Paper 3

Freezing point, melting point, latent heat, vapourisation

Could you define the freezing and boiling points of a substance?

- Freezing point: temperature at which a solid and liquid are in equilibrium at a given pressure; latent heat of fusion
- Boiling point: temperature at which a liquid and its vapour are in equilibrium at a given pressure: latent heat of vapourisation
- Boiling point is very pressure dependent, e.g. desflurane vapouriser, poor cup of tea at altitude!
- Triple point: solid, liquid and vapour in equilibrium: only one combination of pressure and temperature
- SVP: dependence on temperature
- Effect on vapourisers; water vapour at altitude and hypoxia
- N_2O: effect of use on temperature and contents of cylinder
- Critical temperature of N_2O (36.5°C) and O_2 (-119°C)
- N_2O isotherm diagrams
- Colligative properties; freezing point depression, boiling point elevation, osmometers, Raoult's Law, effect on SVP
- Osmolarity, osmolality and isotonic definitions and relevance

Measuring FiO_2 and PO_2

How may the concentration of oxygen in a gas mixture be measured?

- Clark electrode: polarographic cell; 0.6V applied across $Ag/AgCl_2$ – Pt electrode and current flow dependent on O_2 concentration. Gas or liquid: impermeable membrane prevents false high with volatile agents
- Fuel cell: Pb/Au in KOH. O_2 produces EMF. Limited life span, consumed in process, may be affected by N_2O, slow response
- Paramagnetic: O_2 (diatomic) attracted into magnetic field displacing sphere filled with N_2: accurate; null displacement method used in practice
- Mass spectrometer; photoacoustic; Raaman spectroscope
- Chemical: Haldane's apparatus (reduction of volume when oxygen is absorbed by alkaline pyragallol)
- Calibration of blood-gas electrode
- For gas mixtures, PO_2 from FIO_2 and barometric pressure

Pulse oximetry

How does a pulse oximeter work?

What are the sources of inaccuracy – the effect of different haemoglobins?

- Absorption spectroscopy
- Beer-Lambert Law, draw graph, isobestic points, ratio of AC signals
- Low perfusion, ambient light

Paper 4

Physics of gas laws

A partly used size D oxygen cylinder of volume 2.3 L has a pressure of 100 atmospheres. During transport, for how long could it be used to supply oxygen at 4.6 L min^{-1} into a breathing system?

- Volume of O_2 at atmospheric pressure = 2.3 x 100 = 230 L
- time = 230/4.6 = 50 min
- Boyle's Law: PV=const at const T
- Charles' Law: V/T=const at const P (V zero at 0 K)
- Gay-Lussac's Law: P/T= const at const V (P zero at 0 K)
- Universal gas law and constant (PV=nRT)
- Avogadro's hypothesis
- Absolute zero
- Isothermal and adiabatic change (temp rise in air compressor, cooling of cryoprobe)
- Applications of gas laws in anaesthetic practice
- Concept and definition of critical temperature
- Deviations from ideal gas behaviour close to critical temp (use N_2O as example, Tcrit 36.5°C)
- Concept of partial pressures (Dalton's Law)
- Diffusion of gases: principles
- NB some textbooks state that Gay-Lussac's Law is same as Charles' Law

Principles of measurement

What do you understand by the term calibration? What does an ideal calibration curve look like?

- Calibration: comparison of individual measuring device with reference
- Linearity (draw graph: to be certain, needs three points, e.g. FiO_2 at 0%, 21% and 100%)
- Non-linearity (draw graph: often occurs outside calibration range, e.g. pulse oximeter at low SaO_2, oxygen electrode at high PO_2: compensation for non-linearity, e.g. amp of hot wire anemometer
- Signal to noise ratio (mains hum on ECG, diathermy and EEG etc.)
- Artefact: sources and rejection (e.g. flushing of arterial line on displayed values, common mode rejection on ECG, algorithm action/failure on non-invasive blood pressure etc.)
- Drift of zero and gradient (now rare, usually electronic: can be temperature drift in blood gas machine, pressure changes in capnograph chamber)
- Hysteresis. Examples on provided graphs and data given on blood-gas calibration

Breathing systems – Mapleson A, C, D, E and F

Show diagram of different breathing systems. How is efficiency gauged in these breathing systems?

Compare the mechanisms behind the efficiency of some of these systems

- Ratio of carbon dioxide clearance to fresh gas flow
- Describe fresh gas flow in relation to minute volume for spontaneous respiration and IPPV
- Consider cost, pollution, advantages/disadvantages of each system

Paper 5

Capnography

What does a capnometer measure? What are the principles involved in the measurement?

- Infrared beam splits and passes through reference and sample gas chambers
- CO_2 absorbs infrared and emergent beams are compared by either photoelectric cells or by chopping light and reheating CO_2 containing chambers and measuring pressure rise
- Calibrated on air (assumed zero) and known concentration (gas cylinder) or electronically (step input voltage)
- Affected by barometric and extraction pressure in system
- Water vapour trap
- Hygroscopic tubing. Needs N_2O compensation
- Value of capnometry in monitoring and prevention of critical incidents
- (Strictly speaking – capnometer analyses CO_2 and simply displays a numerical figure, capnograph is graphical or trend display)

Bernoulli's principle and Venturi effect

Show the photograph of a ventimask. Can you describe how this works?

- Bernoulli principle, (Bernoulli flow meter), low pressure at constriction, gas velocity and kinetic energy rise: total energy assumed constant so potential energy (pressure) falls
- Entrainment ratio definition
- Peak inspiratory flow rate
- Other applications: nebulisers, injectors, Venturi flow meters
- Density and viscosity of gases
- Choanda effect
- Fluidics

Force, energy and work

What do you understand by 'force' and what are its units?

- Vector: F = m a. Units kg m s^{-2} or Newtons
- Different forms of energy
  - mechanical – kinetic ½ mv^2 and potential mgh
  - thermal – mass x specific heat x temperature change
  - electrical – volts x amps x time
- How are different forms of energy interchanged?
  - mass falls from height
  - motor – electrical into mechanical
  - generator – mechanical into electrical
- What is the relationship between energy and work?
  - Interchangeable both measured in Joules or Nm
  - Work = force x distance = pressure x volume
- What is power and what are its units?
  - Rate of change of energy; J sec^{-1} or Watt

Paper 6

Doppler

Define the Doppler effect, using an equation to help your explanation.

What is duplex Doppler?

What are the medical uses of Doppler?

- Change in received frequency of a sound due to relative motion between sound source and the receiver
- **$V = \Delta F . c / 2F_o . \cos\Theta$**
- Doppler and ultrasound combined, real time colour flow imaging
- Cardiac output monitoring

Cardiac output waveform analysis

What information can be derived from a direct arterial pressure wave?

How can an arterial waveform be used to monitor cardiac output?

- BP, HR, rhythm, cardiac output, fluid responsiveness
- Waveform analysis (calculus), calibration
- Advantages and disadvantages of these devices

Infusion devices

What types of infusion devices are available?

Infusion devices available include:

- Syringe drivers and volumetric pumps
- Errors (show photograph of pump set up with errors)
  - human errors, adequate training
  - anti-reflux valves
  - siphoning
  - alarm settings

Paper 7

Heat loss during anaesthesia and surgery

How is heat lost during anaesthesia and surgery?

Heat is lost in several ways:

- Radiation (40%) – Stefan Bolzmann Law
- Convection (30%)
- Evaporation (15%) – latent heat
- Respiration (10%)
- Conduction (5%)
- Phases of heat loss during general anaesthesia
  - redistribution
  - linear
  - plateau

Methods of reducing heat loss

NICE guidelines

Scavenging systems

What methods are available for reducing the concentration of volatile agents in the theatre atmosphere?

- Don't dwell on asking about alternatives such as TIVA
- Closed circuit (don't dwell on properties of circles)
- Absorption by activated charcoal – not commonly used
- Scavenging: passive and active systems; advantages and disadvantages of each; testing of system
- Possible adverse effects to patients, staff etc.
- Where do the waste gases go?
- Theatre ventilation 15 air changes/h
- Safe limits and national safety standards
- Difficult areas: paediatrics, recovery, obstetrics
- Indications for gas induction

Factors affecting the dynamic response of an arterial line

In what ways may a direct arterial pressure transducer give you false information?

False information may be given as a result of:

- Calibration errors – 1 *vs* 2 *vs* 3 point calibration
- Transducer height – levelling
- Resonance, systems resonant frequency
- Frequency response: Fourier analysis – use of first 10 harmonics
- Damping: optimal and critical
- Phase shift

Paper 8

Heat transfer (using blood as an example)

What are the physical principles involved when blood is warmed prior to transfusion?

- Conduction across tubing wall from water bath/hot plate
- Water bath itself heated by natural convection from hot element: element heated by flow of current through conductor (watts = volts x amps)
- Temperature difference – blood stored at 4°C
- Relevant factors in heat transfer:
  - Surface area
  - Thermal conductivity of plastic tubing
  - Area of contact
  - Speed of flow
- Dangers of hot water baths
- Thermostats and how they work: coefficient of expansion
- Reasons for heat loss (and methods of prevention) during operations
- Core and peripheral temperatures

Electrical hazards

Why is the diathermy pad always checked at the end of an operation?

- Burns and electrical shocks
- Current density
- Skin impedance
- Protective footwear
- Diathermy: frequency and dangers
- Mains supply: live, neutral, earth
- Earth faults, fuses, circuit breakers
- Equipment: class I fully earthed; class II double insulated; class III low voltage
- Macroshock: effects of different amounts of current
- Microshock: causes and effects

Temperature measurement

How may a patient's temperature be measured? What physical principles are involved in the measurement?

- Liquid expansion: large bulb, narrow uniform capillary, lens-shaped wall, clinical thermometer has constriction; low recording design for hypothermia
- Dial: liquid or saturated vapour in Bourdon gauge. Robust, insensitive but not accurate
- Bimetallic strip; cheap, inaccurate
- Chemical: strip of cells filled with mixture of chemicals that melt over a range of temperatures: alternatively, liquid crystals with optical properties dependent on temperature
- Resistance: increases with temperature; Pt, Cu, Ni. Sensitive but fragile instruments
- Thermistor: semi-conductors with resistance that changes with temperature: very small, sensitive: problems with ageing, variability and memory
- Thermocouple Fe/constantan or Cu/constantan (constantan = Cu+Ni). Generates small EMF when heated, so needs sensitive measurement; cold junction at constant temperature or requires compensation

Paper 9

Principles of magnetism

What equipment employs magnets?

Magnets are used in:

- Paramagnetic oxygen analysers, galvanometers, electromagnetic flow meters, mass spectrometers and MRI scanners
- Definition of magnetic flux and magnetic flux density and their units
- Basic principles of an MRI scanner
- Problems with anaesthetising in MRI unit

Measurement of biological potentials

What piece of equipment converts biological signals, measured in microvolts or millivolts, into well-reproduced signals in the order of volts?

- An amplifier (transducer converts physical change, e.g. pressure into another form, e.g. resistance)
- An amplifier makes a recorded change larger so it can be interpreted or passed on more easily. Does not have to be electronic, e.g. lever linkage, microscope
- Electronic: biological and component signals are of very low voltage and need to be made larger before they can be processed or recorded
- Valve: small signal voltage applied to grid controls large changes in anode current
- Transistor: signal applied to base affects flow of current between emitter and collector
- Operational amplifier: very high gain amplifier that produces an output proportional to the difference between its two input voltages
- Advantages: high-input impedance allows high gain without draining source current: differential amplification means interfering signals are rejected (common mode rejection)
- Differential amplifiers. Gain, common mode rejection, frequency response and bandwidth filters

Types of needle used in anaesthetic practice

What types of needle do you use in your anaesthetic practice?

- IV needle (various sizes)
- Short bevel for regional blocks
- Arterial cannulae
- Central venous catheters
- Epidural, spinal needles of various types
- Sanders injector
- Filter needle
- Flow through each – Poiseuille's formula: flow = pressure drop x πr4
- x length x η
- Factors which affect it
- Complications of insertion
- Rapid infusion devices

Paper 10

Electrical components, Ohm's Law, watts, current density

Can you identify the circuit components shown in the diagram?

- If choose resistor: V = I x R, Power = V x I
- Pick other circuit components: how do they work? etc
- DC and AC differences
- Concept of current density and burns (diathermy high frequency constant current, but high current density at probe, low current density at plate)
- Microshock
- Defibrillator circuit and how it works in principle: Coulombs, inductor, Joules, set *vs* delivered energy
- Exponential growth of charge on plates etc.
- Power supplies, Zener diodes etc.

Measurement of cylinder pressure, pressures up to 1 atmosphere, vacuum

If you had to measure the pressure in a gas cylinder, what instrument would you use?

- Cylinders: Bourdon gauge, specialist transducers
- Gauge and absolute pressures in relation to atmosphere
- Various units of pressure measurement
- Aneroid gauge, manometer, barometer, transducers
- Vacuum: definition and uses
- Testing suction, where should it be available?
- Choice of suction catheter and hazards of suction

Disconnection monitors

Which monitors are essential for the induction and maintenance of general anaesthesia?

- Essential: anaesthetist, clinical, SaO_2, ECG, NIBP, $EtCO_2$, FiO_2, vapour, airway pressure, ventilating volumes, PNS and temperature available
- Importance of disconnection as a critical incident. Effects of a disconnection
- Use, advantages and disadvantages of pressure alarms (position in circuit, effect of blocked HME)
- Flow alarms (inspiratory and expiratory)
- FiO_2 meter
- Capnography
- Time response of pulse oximeter to disconnection with high FiO_2
- Limitations of pulse oximeter as a monitor of adequate spontaneous respiration with high inspired FiO_2
- Other information derived from capnograph in addition to disconnection

Notes

Notes